VITAMIN D

*Mr. Seabrook does not author books for fame and glory,
but for the love of writing and sharing his knowledge.*

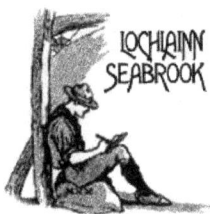

Warning: SEA RAVEN PRESS BOOKS WILL EXPAND YOUR ★ MIND!

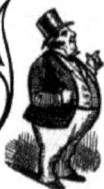

VITAMIN D

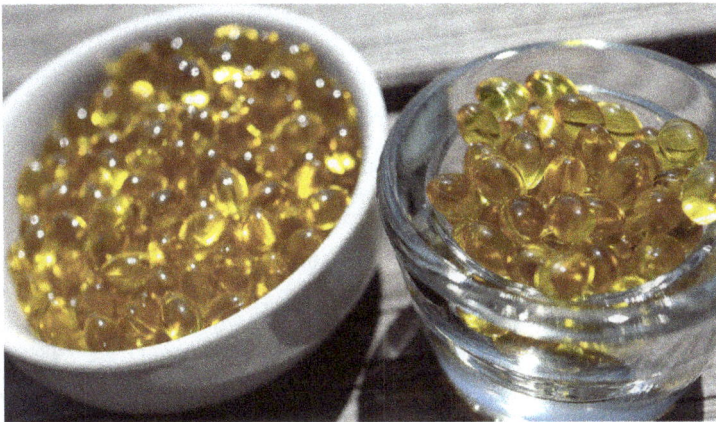

The Miracle Treatment
For Nearly Every Disease And Health Issue

LOCHLAINN SEABROOK

AWARD-WINNING AUTHOR OF *VICTORIAN HERNIA CURES*

Diligently Researched and Generously Illustrated
by the Author for the Elucidation of the Reader

2024

Sea Raven Press, Park County, Wyoming, USA

VITAMIN D

Published by
Sea Raven Press, Cassidy Ravensdale, President
Park County, Wyoming, USA
SeaRavenPress.com

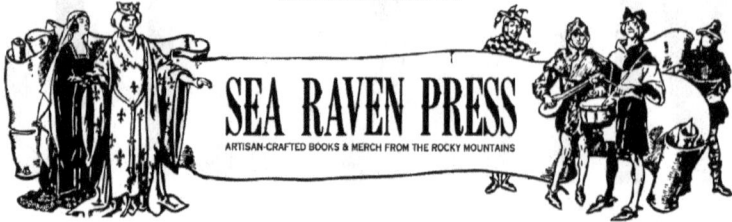

SEA RAVEN PRESS

ARTISAN-CRAFTED BOOKS & MERCH FROM THE ROCKY MOUNTAINS

PRINTING HISTORY
1st SRP paperback edition, 1st printing, August 2024 • ISBN: 978-1-955351-50-8
1st SRP hardcover edition, 1st printing, August 2024 • ISBN: 978-1-955351-48-5

ISBN: 978-1-955351-50-8 (paperback)
Library of Congress Control Number: 2024945686

Vitamin D: The Miracle Treatment for Nearly Every Disease and Health Issue, by Lochlainn Seabrook. Includes an introduction, photographs, illustrations, disclaimer, conversion tables, an index, endnotes, appendices, and a bibliography.

ARTWORK
Front and back cover design and art, book design, layout, font selection, and interior art by Lochlainn Seabrook
All images, image captions, graphic design, and graphic art copyright © Lochlainn Seabrook
All images selected, placed, manipulated, cleaned, colored, tinted, and/or created by Lochlainn Seabrook
Epigraph constructed from Congressional Hearing, p. 727, and Kaplan and Beech, p. 198
Cover and title page photo: "Vitamin D Capsules: The Sunshine Vitamin," by Lochlainn Seabrook

All persons who approve of the authority and principles of Colonel Lochlainn Seabrook's literary work, and realize its benefits as a means of reeducating the world about facts left out of mainstream books, are hereby requested to avidly recommend his titles to others and to vigorously cooperate in extending their reach, scope, and influence around the globe.

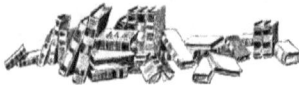

The opinions, theories, & views documented in this book concerning diet and nutrition are those of the publisher.

WRITTEN, DESIGNED, PUBLISHED, PRINTED, & MANUFACTURED IN THE UNITED STATES OF AMERICA

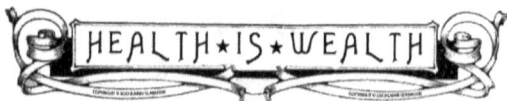

HEALTH ★ IS ★ WEALTH

Dedication

To the fearless pioneers and supporters of vitamin D research.

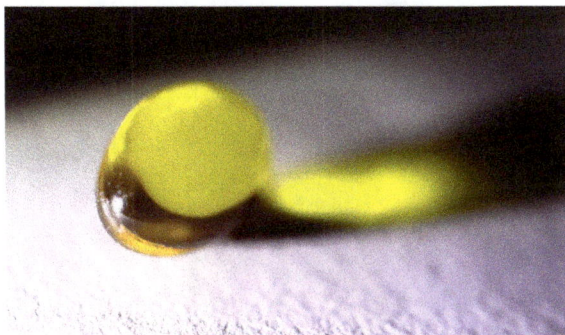

Epigraph

Some 92 percent of Americans are deficient in at least one or more essential vitamin or mineral, "and scientists report that vast numbers of them are suffering from mental and physical sicknesses that simple nutritional solutions might cure."

Hon. Olin E. Teague
Congressional Representative from Texas, 1973

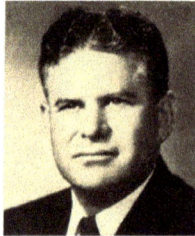

CONTENTS

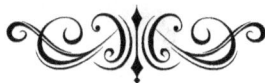

SEA RAVEN PRESS

was founded for the express purpose of publishing and circulating such books as are calculated to store the mind with useful knowledge. We therefore publish only books of a high moral tone and tendency—such works as will be welcomed in every home and at every fireside as valuable family treasures.

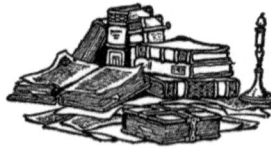

L. SEABROOK

A NOTE TO HEALTHCARE PRACTITIONERS

THE WORLD OF VITAMIN D is a large, complex, often confusing, and ever expanding one, with new discoveries being made about this remarkable compound on an almost daily basis. Contradictions, discrepancies, dissension, heated debate, and passionate opinions, not to mention clinical research that comes to totally opposing conclusions, are rife within the medical community, with no two authorities agreeing on every aspect of vitamin D: what it is, how to get it, what its functions are, how it operates, what it does or does not affect, how to best test it, the proper blood serum level, the correct cell level, or its toxicity levels. There is not even a hint of agreement across the scientific spectrum on how much vitamin D is needed by the average person.

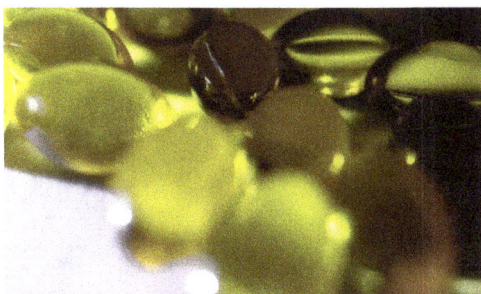

Vitamin D capsules. Photograph by Lochlainn Seabrook. Copyright © Lochlainn Seabrook.

In such a climate, where personal pride and subjective views often hold sway, I have done my level best to make objective sense of this exciting but gargantuan topic, one that holds so much promise for both the individual and the betterment of humanity.

While I have nothing but the highest respect for established medicine and its amazing and dedicated practitioners, admittedly there is still much to learn about vitamin D. No single person, no matter how highly educated, knows all there is to know about it, and no single individual probably ever will. Even at this point, 104 years after its discovery, the subject of vitamin D is simply too vast, with too many variables and obscurities. Not even the actual daily requirement is known yet.

Thus I challenge all medical professionals—both conventional and nonconventional—who read this book to do so with a flexible and inquiring mind. The information it contains is too urgent, important, even earth-shattering. Question everything, yes. Disregard everything, no.

LOCHLAINN SEABROOK

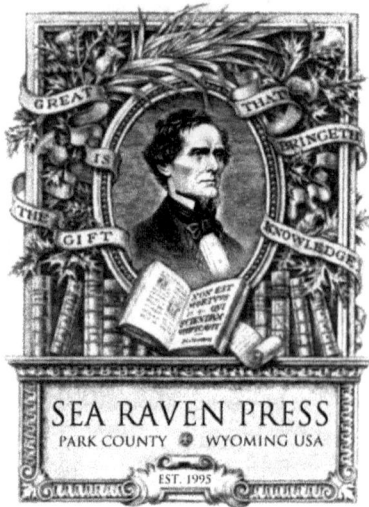

SEA RAVEN PRESS
PARK COUNTY ❧ WYOMING USA

EST. 1995

"Books invite all; they constrain none."
Hartley Burr Alexander (1873-1939)

DISCLAIMER

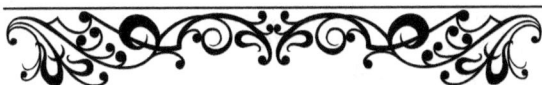

❧ A number of Websites and Webpages are cited in this book. Neither the publisher nor the author are responsible for the availability or content of these sites, nor does the publisher or author endorse, warrant, or guarantee the organizations, businesses, individuals, products, services, or information described or offered on these online sites. In addition, the reader accepts full responsibility for possible risks related to misinformation, disinformation, computer viruses, and copyright and licensing restrictions connected to these Websites.

❧ Neither the publisher nor the author endorse, recommend, or have any connection to, the individuals, organizations, books, papers, studies, Websites, or Webpages, etc., cited in this book.

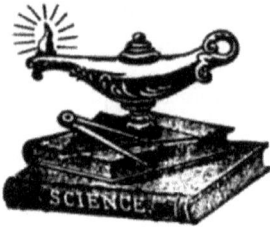

❧ Neither the publisher nor the author has reviewed or evaluated the authenticity, legitimacy, credibility, validity, pertinence, or relevance of any of the individuals or material cited in this book; all individuals, organizations, studies, and materials are cited as found in their original sources. It is up to you the reader to validate or invalidate, as well as form your own judgements relating to, this book's contents.

❧ Because new discoveries are being made, and because new research is being conducted, daily, the reader understands and accepts that some of the information supplied in this book may be, and probably has become, obsolete or proven incorrect or invalid since its writing and publication. Caution is advised.

❧ This book has not been peer-reviewed by the medical, nutritional, or scientific establishment; therefore any and all evaluations, assessments, and conclusions related to statements made by the individuals and material cited in this book are the responsibility of you the reader.

❧ Neither the publisher nor the author assume any obligation or liability—and make no warranties—with respect to the accuracy, usefulness, quality, trustworthiness, or completeness of the information, products, processes, or apparatuses, referred to or described in this book, including what may be obsolete data, inaccuracies, contradictions, typos, errors, opinions, theories, hypotheses, outdated research, etc. It is your responsibility and yours alone to be aware of the above mentioned possible issues as well as determine the value of this book's content.

❧ Warning: Vitamin D is not a vitamin. It is an extremely powerful hormone whose misuse could have dangerous consequences.

❧ Owning, possessing, borrowing, reading, or using this book or its contents in any manner whatsoever infers that you have read, understand, and agree to this Disclaimer and all of the terms and conditions contained therein—without exception. THE PUBLISHER

INTRODUCTION

WRITING THIS BOOK HAS NOT been merely an academic exercise for me. More than anything else it is a public service announcement, a call to action, and a vital health guide focusing on a massive epidemic that is taking place across the globe as I write these words. I am speaking here of what I refer to as *the worldwide vitamin D deficiency pandemic*, a phenomena I only learned about recently—and in a most personal way.

I have always been a robust, outdoorsy, health-conscious individual with a focus on fitness and healthy eating. So it was a great mystery to me why, at the same time, I struggled for many decades with a myriad of often strange and seemingly unrelated health conditions. Mainstream doctors had no idea what was going on, and always fell back on their usual approach to "practicing medicine" by prescribing what I consider largely useless tests, toxic medications, and unnecessary surgeries—none of which, as a lifelong health enthusiast, I was interested in. I believe in preventing disease through long term health maintenance. Established medicine, however, is primarily programmed to do repair work—after the fact.

Some of my ailments have been quite serious, greatly impacting my daily existence in ways that ranged from difficult and uncomfortable to excruciating and even unbearable. Several were life-threatening. I was told by friends and family that it was all part of "aging," while mainstream doctors continued to push the usual bewildering and ponderously massive menu of prescription medicines.

During all of this a thought occasionally crossed my mind: "Is it possible that all of my conditions are connected?" The logical part of my brain rejected the idea outright. "How could they be?" I rationalized to myself. Supporting my doubts, I could find nothing in the medical literature even remotely related to this question.

Years passed. Speculations piled up. New ailments emerged. My suffering increased.

Then, this past spring, through a serendipitous and wholly unaccountable act of Providence, I made a personal discovery that connected all the dots and instantly solved the questions I had surrounding my many seemingly unrelated health problems. The solution I discovered was vitamin D, a so-called "nutrient" that I knew little about at the time. Very rapidly this new knowledge completely changed my life, and immediately put me on the road to recovery. How?

After months of study, hundreds of hours of research, and dozens of self-diagnostic experiments performed on my mind and body, I began to see that the ailments I had been suffering from were indeed interconnected, and that all of them, in fact, stemmed from a *lifelong* and *very severe* vitamin D deficiency. It was this epiphany that prompted me to embark on a treatment regimen of high-dosage vitamin D therapy.

The results have been beyond anything I could have previously imagined. In fact, I began seeing positive changes in my health within only an hour or two of taking my first mega-therapeutic dose. After several weeks, more seemingly miraculous healings followed. Odd and painful conditions I had had, in some cases since early childhood (all are listed in Chapter Three in this book), began to lift, fade, and disappear one by one.

As of this writing my amazing healing transformation continues, with each day bringing new and astounding

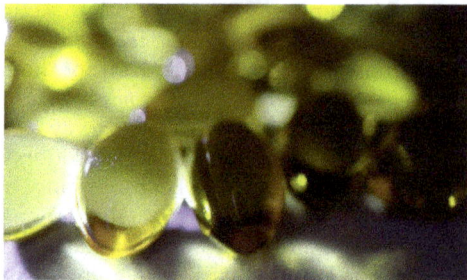

Photograph by Lochlainn Seabrook. Copyright © Lochlainn Seabrook.

results in every area, from energy and mood to the complete eradication of various strange disorders and even a few very significant diseases.

As I looked around me with my new knowledge I realized that nearly everyone I know is also suffering from at least one or more vitamin D deficiency-related illnesses. In other words, depending on your age, weight, skin color, and location, the odds are overwhelmingly high that you yourself are the victim of a vitamin D deficiency. My book, *Vitamin D: The Miracle Treatment for Nearly Every Disease and Health Issue*, is the result of this revelation, written for all those interested in unraveling the mysteries of, and treating, their own health problems.

While it is only meant to be an introduction to the often overwhelming and complex science surrounding vitamin D, this concise amalgamation of my findings is designed to help you discover your own relationship to this potent life-altering chemical—one that can literally make you or break you, depending on your personal knowledge, sense of discipline, intellectual receptivity, and lifestyle.

Open your mind and read on. This information could save your life. It saved mine.

Lochlainn Seabrook
Rocky Mountains, Wyoming
August 2024

CHAPTER 1
UNDERSTANDING VITAMIN D

THE AMERICAN APPROACH TO VITAMIN HEALTH
If you are anything like the average person, when it comes to making sure your body is getting the proper amount of vitamins and minerals, you probably do not give it much thought. Most of us adult Americans, around 75 percent, simply take a few pills every morning, then get on with our busy schedules. The other 25 percent apparently seem to devote no time to thinking about nutrition at all.

The more conscientious may drink a quick glass of orange juice first thing in the morning, or grab an energy bar for lunch. Dinnertime is seen as the one large, "well-rounded" meal of the day, where we assume that we are getting any and all of the nutrients we might have missed at breakfast and lunch.

A great many individuals live their entire lives using this lackadaisical approach to vitamin health—but they do so at their peril, for the body does not merely need, but actually *biologically requires* certain elements to grow, repair itself, and function healthfully and normally on a daily basis. Unfortunately, the average American's understanding of vitamins hinders rather than enhances bodily health, which can lead to a host of consequential problems, as this book will show. Thus it is in one's best interest to have a basic understanding of vitamins, of what they are, how much we need of each one, and the best sources of those vitamins.

THE 13 ESSENTIAL VITAMINS
Currently science recognizes 13 essential vitamins, a number that changes periodically with new research and discoveries. When possible, it is always best to get our vitamins from foods rather than pills, and to eat as wide and varied a diet as possible.

Why is this so important?

Foods contain many nutrients that are not found in vitamin

supplements (this includes a number of mysterious unnamed elements, many which are still unknown, as they have not been discovered yet), but which work together to facilitate digestion and overall good health. Despite their best efforts, scientists have not been able to create vitamins as complete as those formed naturally by Mother Nature and which she has gifted to us as "food." So the wise get as many of their nutrients as possible from a wide variety of meats, dairy products, grains, fruits, vegetables, nuts, and seeds. The ancient Greek philosopher Hippocrates wisely said: "Let food be your medicine," an axiom that, as you will see, forms part of the very foundation of this book.

What follows are the common and scientific names of the 13 essential vitamins, along with their primary *food* sources:

Vitamin A (retinol): dairy, vegetables, fruits.
Vitamin B1 (thiamine): meat, grains.
Vitamin B2 (riboflavin): eggs, meat, vegetables.
Vitamin B3 (niacin): legumes, grains, nuts, meat.
Vitamin B5 (pantothenic acid): meat, grains, vegetables, dairy.
Vitamin B6 (pyridoxine): meat, starchy vegetables, fruit.
Vitamin B7 (niacin): meat, eggs, nuts, seeds, avocados.
Vitamin B9 (folate): vegetables, fruits, nuts, legumes.
Vitamin B12 (cobalamin): meat, dairy.
Vitamin C (ascorbic acid): fruits, vegetables.
Vitamin D (calciferol): fish (oils).
Vitamin E (alpha-tocopherol): nuts, oils, green vegetables.
Vitamin K1 (phylloquinone): green leafy vegetables, fruit, eggs, cheese, meat. (Also includes vitamin K2, menaquinone-7, primarily of bacterial origin.)

It is clear from this simplified list alone that eating a restricted diet, like veganism, can severely impact one's chances for optimal health.[1] It is not that it cannot be done, only that the greatest care must be taken to get the proper amount of each essential nutrient.[2]

Why are these 13 nutrients called "essential" vitamins? Because our bodies need them to function normally and because our bodies cannot manufacture enough of them to meet our daily requirements. This means that in order to maintain health, essential vitamins must be procured from sources outside our bodies.[3]

THE EXISTENTIAL VITAMIN

The most important vitamin in the list above, the one *most* important to your overall health, to your very mental and physical existence, is one you will almost never notice, never see highlighted on TV or the Internet, never hear discussed by doctors on health panels. Mainstream doctors seldom, if ever, mention vitamin D, and not even conventional nutritionists themselves devote much time to this mysterious chemical.

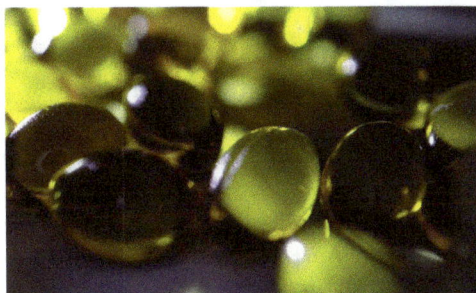

Photograph by Lochlainn Seabrook. Copyright © Lochlainn Seabrook.

Such attitudes would seem to infer that it is a vitamin of little importance, that it is easily obtained, and that little thought need be given it. Indeed, many established health practitioners actually preach this very thing.

All of this could not be more wrong, *and* dangerous!

In discussing the master vitamin D, I am speaking of an element so omnipotent, so vitally essential to both quality of life and life itself, that I have nicknamed it "the existential vitamin," and have dedicated this entire book to it—for reasons which will become increasingly clear.

WHAT IS VITAMIN D?

Discovered in the period from 1918 to 1922 during an intense scientific search for a cure for the childhood bone disease known as rickets,[4] the dictionary defines vitamin D as:

> "Any or all of several fat-soluble vitamins chemically related to steroids, essential for normal bone and tooth structure, and found especially in fish-liver oils, egg yolk, and milk, or produced by activation (as by ultraviolet irradiation) of sterols."[5]

Science actually currently identifies five different forms of vitamin D:

1. Vitamin D1: A molecular compound of ergocalciferol and lumisterol.
2. Vitamin D2: Ergocalciferol (derives from plant products).
3. Vitamin D3: Cholecalciferol (derives from animal products).
4. Vitamin D4: Dihydrotachysterol (dihydroergocalciferol).
5. Vitamin D5: Sitocalciferol.

There are only two *authentic, natural, health-giving* forms of vitamin D, however, and these are vitamin D2 (considered by alternative health practitioners to be less effective than, and thus inferior to, D3)[6] and vitamin D3, the latter being the subject of this work.[7] The other three types of vitamin D (1, 4, and 5) are chemically altered synthetic forms with questionable health benefits.[8] Thus, unless I state otherwise, *all* references I make to "vitamin D" in the following pages specifically apply to vitamin D3 and only to vitamin D3.

THE MECHANISMS & FUNCTIONS OF VITAMIN D3

Vitamin D3 plays dozens if not hundreds of roles in human health, so many, in fact, that we are not yet aware of all of them, with many being only newly discovered, and more amazing findings being made on an almost monthly basis.

Its most important function, however, is the creation, building, and maintenance of strong healthy bones[9] and cartilage (which prompted the original research in the 1920s).[10] New evidence reveals that vitamin D3 is probably more important than calcium (one of the "anti-toxin minerals")[11] for maintaining bone integrity and density, for vitamin D not only promotes calcium absorption (more than calcium intake itself does),[12] but it also helps bones store calcium longer, which lowers one's risk of fractures and other bone-related issues and diseases.[13]

Though now outdated in some respects, the following 51 year old description of the functions of vitamin D comes from the U.S. government:

"Regulates the use of calcium and phosphorus in the body and is therefore necessary for the proper formation of teeth and bones. Very important in infancy and childhood to prevent rickets. Vitamin D is called the sunshine vitamin as it is produced by the action of sunlight on a substance secreted by the oil glands of the skin. It aids in the healing of fractured bones. Vitamin D should not be taken in excessive doses. It has been used in treating arthritis by some doctors. It may have a good effect on liver action."[14]

Even more important to our understanding of vitamin D than its many functions, however, is the fact that it is not a "vitamin" at all, but rather an anti-inflammatory, antimicrobial, antiviral *hormone*[15] that is responsible for, regulates, or contributes to:

• Calcium absorption—augmenting bone health (as noted).
• Phosphorus absorption—augmenting protein, bone, and tissue regulation and health.
• Immune function—augmenting autoimmune health.
• Gene expression, gene repair, and gene stability—augmenting molecular and genetic health.
• Cerebral stability—augmenting brain health.
• Mental stability—augmenting psychological health.
• Musculature strength—augmenting muscle health.
• Cell differentiation and proliferation (apoptosis), as well as cell production—augmenting cellular health.
• Defense against viral and bacterial infections—augmenting overall biological health.
• Neurogenesis—augmenting nervous system health.
• Inflammation control—augmenting organ health.

This little list covers nearly *every* cell, tissue, structure, organ, and system in the body,[16] affecting our health in a wide variety of ways that manifest, as we shall see, in over 1,000 diseases and health conditions that I have uncovered—all preventable, treatable, or associated with vitamin D in some manner.

THE SCIENCE BEHIND VITAMIN D
Vitamin D is actually a term referring to an entire group of

chemicals that come from cholesterol, with the two primary forms being the *inactive* vitamin D2 (also known as calciferol or ergocalciferol),[17] which is derived from plants, and the *active* vitamin D3 (cholecalciferol), which comes from animal products. Being passive forerunners of substances formed in, or necessary for, metabolism (known as metabolites), neither diet-derived vitamin D2 or diet-derived vitamin D3 are truly "vitamins," but rather hormones. To this same category must be added 7-dehydrocholesterol, a chemical in the skin that produces cholecalciferol when exposed to sunlight.[18] Additionally, it is important to know that the body handles the work of synthesizing, assimilating, and activating vitamin D through two primary systems: the endocrine system and the paracrine and intercrine system.[19]

Here is how it all works.

After being absorbed (either through the skin or via ingestion), calciferol and cholecalciferol are carried to the liver where they are transmuted to another chemical known as calcidiol (25-hydroxyvitamin D). During the next step in the process, calcidiol attaches to blood proteins, then travels to the kidneys, where it is altered to yet another powerful derivative of vitamin D: calcitriol (1,25-dihydroxyvitamin D).[20]

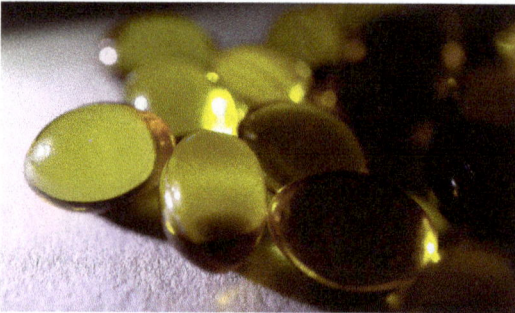

Photograph by Lochlainn Seabrook. Copyright © Lochlainn Seabrook.

These seemingly trivial microscopic processes are essential not only to health, but to life itself. In a biomedical paper entitled "Physiological Basis for Using Vitamin D to Improve Health," Sunil J. Wimalawansa writes that vitamin D is absolutely essential for life, for it is responsible for metabolism, immune functions, and hormonal release,[21] arguably three of the most vital physical processes that take place in our bodies.

He further states that both the active enzyme responsible for synthesizing vitamin D, along with its vitamin D receptors (VDRs), are omnipresent in the body's cells,[22] where they regulate the expression of some 2,700 different genes[23] (13.5 percent of a total of 20,000 genes), while simultaneously adjusting both physiological and metabolic activities.[24] Let us note here that "VDRs are active in virtually all tissues." These include including the kidney, lung, ovary, colon, bone, breast, pancreatic b-cells, melanocytes, keratinocytes, monocytes, parathyroid gland, T lymphocytes, and also cancer cells.[25]

In simplest terms then, vitamin D3—the form we are focusing on—is a secosteroid hormone that, which, while it can be found in small amounts in certain animal foods, is mainly produced endogenously (that is, within the body) by exposure to UVB rays (sunlight), which trigger vitamin D synthesis.[26]

The vitamin D thus produced (or ingested in foods or supplements) is picked up by VDRs, the vitamin D3 receptors, that are found in every cell and tissue in our body,[27] demonstrating the all-important universal nature of, as well as the body-wide functions performed by this misnamed though utterly remarkable royal hormone: vitamin D.[28]

Let me paraphrase and repeat this last statement, for it is one of the most important facts in this entire book: *Every cell in your body is programmed to detect, absorb, and work with the hormone known as "vitamin D."*

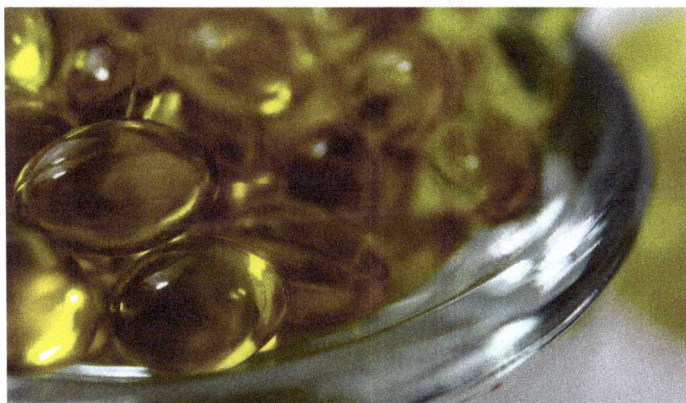

Photograph by Lochlainn Seabrook. Copyright © Lochlainn Seabrook.

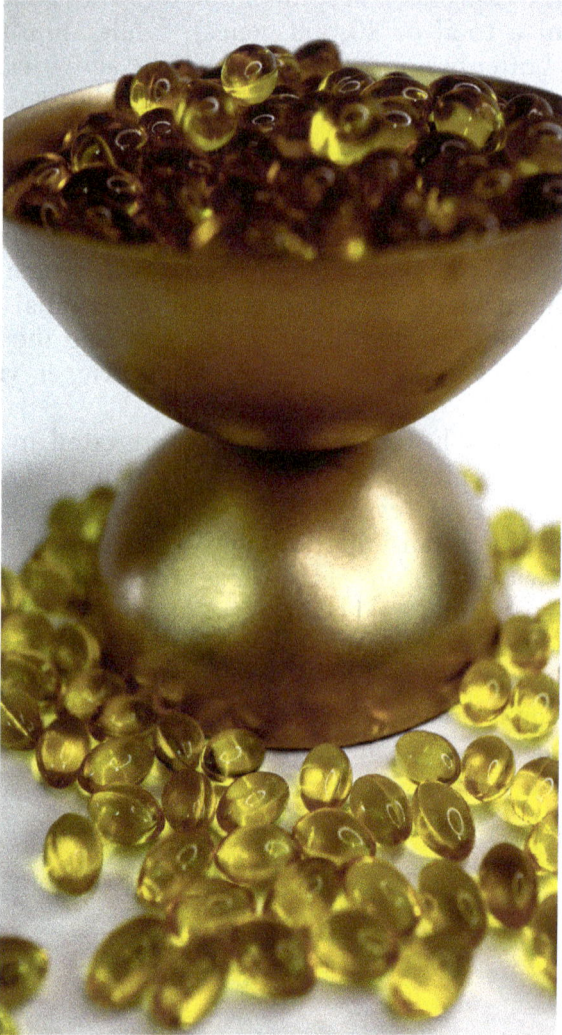

Photograph by Lochlainn Seabrook. Copyright © Lochlainn Seabrook.

CHAPTER 2
RDA, SOURCES, & TESTING

THE MAINSTREAM MEDICAL RDA
In part, because it is still relying on outdated childhood rickets research from the 1920s,[29] the U.S. government, like most other conventional sources today, is grossly under-prescribing the "recommended dietary allowance" (RDA) for vitamin D3.[30] As late as 1973 the U.S. government was still pushing a paltry RDA of just 400 IU for everyone from "the breast-fed baby" to adults,[31] even going as far as to state absurdly:

> "Healthy adults receiving adequate diets *have no need for supplementary vitamins* except during pregnancy and lactation when 400 U.S.P. units of vitamin D daily are required."[32]

During a heated discussion at a 1973 congressional hearing before the House of Representatives, a woman was quoted as saying that "taking vitamins at the U.S. RDA level had no more effect on her than taking a glass of water."[33] In other words, our government's recommended dietary allowances for vitamins are so low that most health-conscious people find them virtually unnoticeable and therefore completely useless.

Nonetheless, so my readers can make their own educated decision regarding the current U.S. RDA, I provide it here:

AGE	MALE	FEMALE	PREGNANCY	LACTATION
0-12 months	400 IU	400 IU		
1-13 years	600 IU	600 IU		
14-18 years	600 IU	600 IU	600 IU	600 IU
19-50 years	600 IU	600 IU	600 IU	600 IU
51-70 years	600 IU	600 IU		
>70 years	800 IU	800 IU[34]		

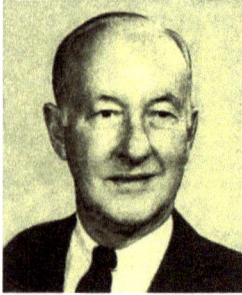

Rep. Charles M. Teague.

At this point it should be stressed that from the very beginning the FDA's "nutritional tyranny"[35] in setting the vitamin D RDA so low, not to mention its attempt to have vitamin D labeled a "prescription-only drug," was met by fierce opposition from the public. After the 1973 hearing just referenced, California Republican Representative Charles M. Teague said:

"It becomes necessary to examine the question of whether or not the implementation of these new regulations is valid from a scientific viewpoint. In the noticeable lack of circulation with respect to the magnitude of contradictory and opposing testimony that occurred at the hearing, the FDA has been misleading Congress and the public. [The] FDA 'Findings of Fact' does not reflect nor incorporate much of that testimony contrary to their original attitudes. As it were, 11 opposition expert witnesses testified that the RDA (recommended daily [dietary] allowance) was never intended to be incorporated into rigid laws governing and limiting the diet patterns for safe nutrients desired by consumers, and that it should not now be used for this purpose.

". . . There is at present insufficient knowledge of the requirements for various nutrients upon which to base such rigid and prohibitive regulations, and that since the science of nutrition changes so rapidly there is always a time lag involved in revising a standard of identity once it becomes effective. A number of opposing witnesses testified to this.

"Additionally, the FDA has evidently not given sufficient weight to several aspects of this matter, i.e., to the deterioration of the eating habits of the American people; to widespread deficiencies in several vitamins which have consistently shown up in all nutrition surveys in the United States to date; and to the fact that 29 experts testified that the RDA is not adequate for substantial numbers of the population."[36]

"Not adequate" indeed.

The frustrations surrounding this issue eventually came

to a boil, and at some point (presumably in the early 2000s), the *mainstream* Institute of Medicine (IOM), now known as the National Academy of Medicine (NAM), raised its own RDA for vitamin D from 400 IU (10 mcg) a day to 2,000 IU (50 mcg) a day[37]—which the medical establishment considers the "upper-limit" safe dose.[38] One other *mainstream* source I came across now recommends between 1,000 IU (25 mcg) to 5,000 IU (125 mcg) as a daily maintenance dose.[39]

But, as we shall see, in almost every case even these dosages are still below what the body actually needs, particularly those under stress, those with severe illnesses, or those with an extreme vitamin D deficiency—or what is known medically as *hypovitaminosis D*. In fact, the original RDA of 400 daily IU for adults is barely enough to prevent rickets and other bone diseases; it is certainly not anywhere near the amount needed to create and sustain optimal health.

The conflict between these two disparate views continues, and it has today become so intense that some enlightened doctors now believe it is time to demand that the U.S. government substantially raise the RDA for vitamin D.[40]

THE ALTERNATIVE MEDICAL RDA
Now let us look at the other side of the coin: The alternative, naturopathic, or nonconventional field of medicine, as it is variously called.

Health practitioners from this group maintain that it is not only safe but absolutely necessary to consume at least 5,000 to 10,000 IU (250 mcg) of vitamin D a day.[41] According to these individuals the 600 to 800 IU now recommended by mainstream medicine is simply too modest to create and maintain everyday health, let alone peak health. And while mainstream doctors argue that anything over 1,000 IU can be toxic, natural doctors cite numerous studies demonstrating that taking 10,000 IU of vitamin D every day is perfectly safe,[42] that "it is very hard to overdose on vitamin D,"[43] and that because of this, vitamin D overloading is "extremely rare," with most doctors never encountering a single instance of toxicity (known medically as *hypervitaminosis D*)[44]—even in one case where an individual took 150,000 IU (3,750 mcg) of vitamin D a day for two years.[45]

To prove the point, as an experiment one scientist took a therapeutic dose of between 25,000 (625 mcg) and 100,000 IU (2,500 mcg) of vitamin D3 daily for over one year. The result? Not only did he *not* suffer from any type of vitamin D toxicity, *all* of his health issues—many which he had had for years—disappeared.[46]

Using what is known as the "Coimbra Protocol," a Brazilian MD, Dr. Cicero Coimbra, treats patients with autoimmune diseases using between 40,000 (1,000 mcg) and 300,000 IU (7,500 mcg) of vitamin D3 a day. According to reports, Dr. Coimbra witnessed "r e m a r k a b l e" improvements in nearly all of his patients, with many of them finding themselves "completely free" of any and all

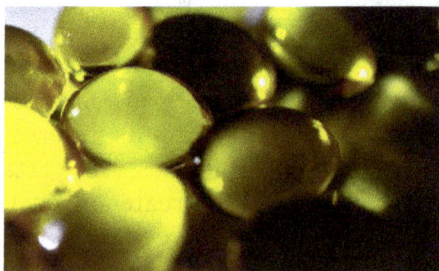

Photograph by Lochlainn Seabrook. Copyright © Lochlainn Seabrook.

symptoms and manifestations of their former diseases.[47]

A 2014 medical paper entitled "Large, Single-dose, Oral Vitamin D Supplementation in Adult Populations: A Systematic Review," noted that the mainstream RDA is usually insufficient when trying to correct a vitamin D deficiency, and that a "single, large dose of vitamin D, given at timed intervals," is more likely to obtain the desired results.[48] After studying 2,243 Pub Med articles related to "high dose vitamin D," this same panel recommended that supplemental vitamin D3 be used over vitamin D2, and concluded that single vitamin D3 doses of 300,000 IU or more "are most effective."[49]

In another case an individual took 500,000 (12,500 mcg) IU of vitamin D for two years without ill effect.[50] An in-depth, nine-year, 1928 study that involved hundreds of doctors and nearly 1,000 patients, looked into the question of vitamin D toxicity. Known as the Steck Report, it found that a 110 lb. woman could safely take up to 1 million IU (25,000 mcg) of vitamin D per day for "indeterminate lengths of time." Several individuals in the study were given 200,000 IU (5,000 mcg) of vitamin D a day for seven years. No deaths occurred. One of the doctors involved in the study experimented on himself by taking 3 million IU (75,000 mcg) of vitamin D a day for 15 days "without any evidence of disturbance of any kind."[51]

In fact, it is believed by many nutritional authorities that all of the few known actual cases of "vitamin D toxicity" can be accounted for by one of the following reasons:

"1. The use of synthetic vitamin D, as reported by Dr. Weston Price and others.[52]
"2. The use of vitamin D alone as a medicine, and without the support of other necessary nutrients [now called "co-factors"]. It is well known that vitamin D is metabolized better when it is supported by the rest of the health team, especially vitamin A, choline, and linoleic acid (from unsaturated oils).
"3. Vitamin D may not be properly utilized in the body when some of the glands or other organs are diseased."[53]

What then is the everyday natural health, or alternative medicine, *maintenance* RDA for vitamin D?

A general recommendation, depending on the current vitamin D level in one's body (see "Testing Blood Levels" below), would be an RDA of 1,000 IU (25 mcg) of vitamin D3 for every 20 lbs. of body weight.[54] According to this formula-ratio, a 100 lb. individual would take 5,000 IU of vitamin D3 a day; a 200 lb. individual would take 10,000 IU a day.[55]

A more aggressive approach, and one used *without any toxicity issues* by at least one notable physician, recommends 30,000 IU per day as a maintenance dose, with an optimal blood level of vitamin D3 of 100-140 ng/ml. While this may seem extraordinarily high to some, please bear in mind that when converted to micrograms, 30,000 IU of D3 is the equivalent of 750 mcg,[56] which is itself a mere 0.75 mg.

A more conservative (and some would say safer) alternative RDA for everyone—from one year of age to seniors—would be 1,500 (37.5 mcg) IU per day[57]—although it must be said that this number is far below the amount at which most individuals can detect any "noticeable positive effects" from taking supplemental vitamin D3.[58]

A natural followup question must be: What is the natural health, or alternative medicine, *therapeutic* RDA for vitamin D; that is for those with either a severe vitamin D deficiency or those suffering from vitamin D-related illnesses?

Here the advice is less specific since high dosage vitamin D therapy is more individualistic—and, according to orthodox medicine, riskier. For severely deficient cases, however, the general practice is around 7,000 IU per day (or 50,000 IU per week) for eight weeks,[59] after which the individual is returned to the normal maintenance dosage of one of the RDAs described above.

At this time there is no agreement among scientists, doctors, or nutritionists concerning either the proper RDA or the actual toxicity level of vitamin D3. Neither measure, in fact, is precisely known yet,[60] which, as we have seen, is partly why the opinions and views regarding these two subjects vary wildly from one extreme to the other. Thus, in either case, whether one chooses to follow a maintenance RDA or a therapeutic RDA of vitamin D, mainstream or alternative, always do so under the care and guidance of your doctor, who will put you on a personalized program that fits your specific health needs.

THE GREAT VITAMIN D COVERUP
From the examples above it is clear that high dosages of vitamin D are not normally toxic, but, under the proper professional guidance, are actually both corrective and even curative.

There is yet another problem with the conventional RDA, however. Depending on your skin color, age, weight, location (latitude), the season, and the air quality where you live, on average, being in the sun for just 12 minutes can synthesize 3,000 IU (75 mcg) of vitamin D3 inside your body,[61] while getting sun exposure for 30 to 40 minutes can generate up to as much as 20,000 IU (500 mcg).[62] Thus the skin *naturally* generates about 34 times more vitamin D than the conventional RDA promoted by the U.S. government and mainstream science. What does this tell us?

Mother Nature herself reveals that established orthodox medicine is far off the mark when it comes to its daily recommended dietary allowance of 600 IU of vitamin D for middle-aged adults.

Why are we being lied to by the mainstream medical establishment?[63] Why has the pharmaceutical industry ("Big Pharma") been gaslighting the public for decades about vitamin D?[64] Why, in the early 1970s, did the Food and Drug Administration, the FDA, try to "arbitrarily" classify vitamin D as a "drug," force it to be sold "by prescription only," then attempt to set a legal limit of 400 IU on the vitamin—all against the will of Congress and the majority of American citizens?[65] And why have thousands of vitamin D deficient hospital patients been allowed to die over the years in what some doctors have angrily described as "FDA murder"?[66]

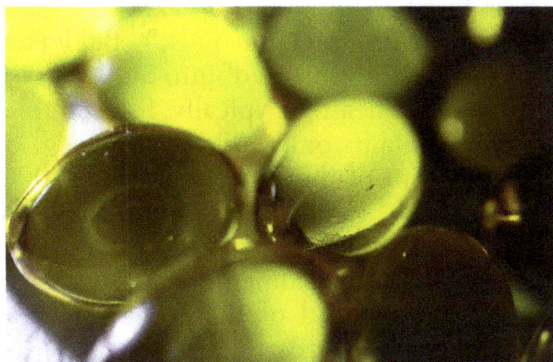

Photograph by Lochlainn Seabrook. Copyright © Lochlainn Seabrook.

The most probable answer to all these questions is, partly at least, financial greed.[67] Vitamin D, in the form of sunlight, is *free*, *non-patentable*, and *easily accessible* to anyone, who can then treat their own illnesses—and in many cases even cure themselves of nearly every known disease (outside those caused by natural aging)—without any reliance on doctors, medications, or surgery.

To combat this particular "problem," the medical establishment invented "new" drugs, like Deltatin, Viosterol, and Drisdol, which are nothing more than high dosages (e.g., 50,000 IU) of vitamin D, often masquerading as cancer-fighting prescription medications.[68] In this way, patients are duped into paying for something that is either already free (vitamin D from sunlight) or relatively inexpensive in comparison (vitamin D from food and supplements).[69]

Some conspiracy theorists have even postulated that the government is using what I call "the Great Vitamin D Coverup" as a means of keeping down American population numbers. I will let you decide if these views have any truth behind them or not.

FOOD SOURCES OF VITAMIN D

Not surprisingly for a vitamin whose primary source is sunlight, the amount of vitamin D necessary to sustain maximum health can be difficult to acquire—which is why it has long been added to foods in the form of "fortified vitamin D."[70] In fact, according to one establishment source, "fortified foods [such as fortified milk and breakfast cereals] provide most of the vitamin D in American diets."[71] But let us note that the vitamin D artificially "fortified" into our foods is nowhere near enough to sustain health. Typically, for example, one cup of fortified milk contains only 100 IU (2.5 mcg) of vitamin D,[72] a mere 1 percent of the approximately 10,000 IU (250 mcg) of vitamin D3 the average adult seems to need each day. Additionally, food manufacturers tend to use vitamin D2 (an inferior form that is often human-made, and thus inactive, rather than natural) instead of the far stronger and more effective vitamin D3, to fortify their products.[73]

While we cannot hope to get enough vitamin D from any single source, and in particular from food alone, it is wise to be aware of which foods have the most vitamin D3. Below is a list I have compiled of the top ten *natural, non-fortified* food sources for vitamin D, in order of their potency:

1. Cod liver oil (highest).
2. Trout.
3. Salmon.
4. Shiitake, portabella, and white mushrooms (need to be grown in the sun, or receive sun exposure).
5. Sardines.
6. Eggs.
7. Beef liver.
8. Tuna fish.
9. Cheddar and Edam cheese.
10. Ground beef (lowest).[74]

The primary difficulty with even these vitamin D-rich foods is that one simply cannot eat enough of them to get an adequate daily amount of vitamin D.[75] Another issue: In many regions of the world these particular foods are unknown, or they are rare or expensive, or both.

As far as deriving adequate vitamin D from food in general, we must consider that most of the foods people eat today are highly processed (heated, denatured, irradiated, chemicalized, bleached, etc.); meaning that what little natural nutrients were in them to begin with have been stripped away—this includes, of course, vitamin D3, not to mention its co-factors, such as magnesium (another "anti-toxin mineral"),[76] calcium, and vitamin K2 (more on these momentarily).

Here we have just a few of the reasons why so many people are deficient in vitamin D today.

SUNLIGHT AS A SOURCE OF VITAMIN D

There is one source of vitamin D, however, that is not in real shortage anywhere in the world, and that is sunlight—making it the best and, for the most part, the most reliable and efficacious source, and the reason for which it is often called "the sunshine vitamin." Since humans evolved outdoors—with our earliest ancestors spending some 12 hours a day in sunlight from birth to death—it is not surprising to learn that to this day sunshine makes up to 90 percent of the average person's annual intake of vitamin D.[77]

According to the National Institutes of Health (NIH), a mainstream U.S. government body that describes itself as "the largest biomedical research agency in the world"[78]:

> "Most people in the world meet at least some of their vitamin D needs through exposure to sunlight. Type B UV (UVB) radiation with a wavelength of approximately 290–320 nanometers penetrates uncovered skin and converts cutaneous 7-dehydrocholesterol to previtamin D3, which in turn becomes vitamin D3. Season, time of day, length of day, cloud cover, smog, skin melanin content, and sunscreen are among the factors that affect UV radiation exposure and vitamin D synthesis. Older people and people with dark skin are less able to produce vitamin

D from sunlight. UVB radiation does not penetrate glass, so exposure to sunshine indoors through a window does not produce vitamin D.

"The factors that affect UV radiation exposure, individual responsiveness, and uncertainties about the amount of sun exposure needed to maintain adequate vitamin D levels make it difficult to provide guidelines on how much sun exposure is required for sufficient vitamin D synthesis. Some expert bodies [organizations] and vitamin D researchers suggest, for example, that approximately 5-30 minutes of sun exposure, particularly between 10 a.m. and 4 p.m., either daily or at least twice a week to the face, arms, hands, and legs without sunscreen usually leads to sufficient vitamin D synthesis. Moderate use of commercial tanning beds that emit 2% to 6% UVB radiation is also effective."[79]

Unfortunately, even in places where sunshine is abundant, not everyone gets enough sunlight. Sometimes tropical climates are too hot and humid for individuals to spend quality time outdoors; thus even countries like Brazil, which sits directly on the equator, can have extremely high rates of vitamin D deficiency.[80] At the other end of the spectrum, for much of the year boreal regions can be too cold for sunbathing. Then we have infants, the sick, and the infirm, all groups that, for good reason, tend to remain indoors.

The elderly are also usually known to get less sun than the young, but this need not be. *The sun is free*, and seniors, wherever they live, can just as easily access the light from our nearest star as those half their age. This is particularly important when one realizes that those over age 70 have half the ability to make vitamin D from sunlight as when they were younger[81]—an important fact for seniors to keep in mind.

THE FABRICATED FEAR: HELIOPHOBIA

One excuse for avoiding the sun is fear of skin cancer, and little wonder. Our own government refers to UV radiation (sunlight) as a "carcinogen," and strongly recommends limiting exposure to the sun's rays.[82] From every direction we are advised to "stay out of the sun," and when this is not possible, to wear sunglasses, long-sleeved shirts, long dresses, and high-SPF sunblock, anything to guard against the "toxic" rays of our solar neighbor.[83]

This unwarranted paranoia began in the 1970s and 1980s when the American Medical Association (AMA), working in tandem with the avaricious cosmetic industry, began issuing bogus warnings to the public regarding "the dangers of sunlight," and the need to wear some type of chemical sunblock—which they then began adding to their products in order to increase sales.[84]

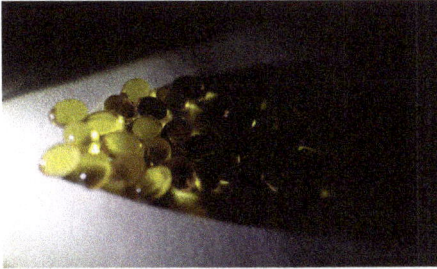

Photograph by Lochlainn Seabrook. Copyright © Lochlainn Seabrook.

Ever since the creation of this manufactured fear, diseases and health issues connected to vitamin D deficiency, as well as the near complete avoidance of an outdoor life, have risen astronomically—along with obesity from lack of exercise.[85]

There is a tremendous amount of debate surrounding the topics of sunlight, UVB radiation, sunscreen, and sun exposure, all of which fall outside the scope of this introductory guide to vitamin D. What I will say on the matter, beyond which there is no dispute, is that heliophobia (fear of the sun) is illogical, unhealthy, and unscientific.

Why? Because it is obvious, from all the evidence, that humans were designed (by God/Nature) to live and work in the sun, for we possess the perfect biological mechanisms for absorbing and transmuting sunlight into vitamin D.[86] We cannot, for example overdose on vitamin D from sunlight (there are no recorded cases of vitamin D toxicity from overexposure to sunlight.)[87] Thus, by avoiding going outside, by constantly hiding away from the sun, by blocking it with clothing and sunscreen when we do venture out, we are short-circuiting our body's built-in natural system for creating and maintaining health.

The general consensus among today's natural health professionals is straightforward: Mainstream medicine has long overplayed the dangers of sunlight,[88] and, providing you do not have a susceptibility to or a history of skin cancer, a judicious amount of sunbathing (not to be confused with tanning) without sunscreen—and with exposure of the face, arms, abdomen, back, hands, and legs in the early morning and/or late afternoon sun—is not only acceptable but desirable when it comes to avoiding vitamin D deficiency.[89]

Indeed, people who live in high sun areas tend to live longer, for their bodies are more easily able to make the active, healthiest, and most important form of vitamin D: vitamin D3. And those with the highest levels of vitamin D3 in their blood not only tend to live the longest, they also tend to have the healthiest quality lives.[90]

Note that applying sunscreen inhibits your body's ability to synthesize vitamin D, which spotlights the importance of getting sunscreen-free early morning and/or late afternoon sun—when its rays are least harmful.[91] (As mentioned above, some authorities recommend the opposite; namely, sunbathing between 10:00 AM and 4:00 PM. Decide what is best for your individual needs.)

When getting real sun is not practical or possible, however, ultraviolet sunlamps and tanning beds can be used as adjuncts for getting vitamin D. (Caveat: There are those who question the benefits of tanning beds since they give out not only beneficial vitamin D-creating UVB rays, but also skin-damaging UVA rays.)[92]

SUPPLEMENTS AS A SOURCE OF VITAMIN D
Due to the many issues involved with getting sufficient vitamin D, most of us must turn to vitamin D supplements. As long as the vitamins are natural (not synthetic)[93] and food-based (that is, derived from real, preferably organic, foods), and do not contain toxic additives, fillers, coloring, and preservatives, this appears to be an ideal solution to this global epidemic.

WHEN & HOW TO TAKE VITAMIN D SUPPLEMENTS
There is an optimal time and manner in which to take vitamin D3. Because vitamin D is a fat-soluble hormone, one that educated doctors more correctly refer to as "hormone D,"[94] it only breaks down in the presence of fat. Thus, you should always take vitamin D with a fatty meal, something, for example, that includes meat, dairy, nuts, or avocados. Taking

it without fat, or even worse, on an empty stomach, is simply a waste of time and money, since most of it will be carried out of the body rather than properly absorbed.

A few doctors recommend taking vitamin D in the morning, when your body most needs energy replenishment to begin the day. However, if you do not eat breakfast, or if you are a vegan who eats a low-fat diet, you should wait to take your vitamin D until your largest and most fat-rich meal—usually dinner.

CO-FACTORS THAT HELP INCREASE VITAMIN D ABSORPTION

Nothing occurs in a vacuum, particularly one's health; thus we should always assume that there are many factors at work affecting our health. To ensure maximum health benefits then, this means that we must approach vitamin D therapy in a *wholistic* manner.

To begin with, a number of studies strongly suggest that the potency and bioavailability of vitamin D are both greatly enhanced by taking it with several co-factors, mainly magnesium glycinate and vitamin K2 (menaquinone-7, or MK-7).[95] Again, one should take all three supplements *simultaneously* during the same high-fat meal, for some studies show that it can actually be dangerous to ingest therapeutic dosages of vitamin D without these two co-factors—one of the greatest risks being the development of hypercalcemia.[96]

Other co-factors that seem to help increase the absorption and activity of vitamin D are:

Boron.
Calcium.
Omega 3.
Probiotics.
Stress management.
Vigorous exercise.
Vitamin A.
Zinc.[97]

In order to safely work these co-factors into your health regimen discuss them with your doctor.

THE VITAMIN D3 & CO-FACTOR RDA FORMULA

How much vitamin K2 and magnesium should an average adult take in relation to the amount of daily vitamin D3?

The recommended *daily* formula-ratio for the alternative medical maintenance RDA for vitamin D3 and its two primary co-factors is as follows:

Vitamin D3: 10,000 IU (250 mcg).
Vitamin K2: 100 mcg.[98]
Magnesium glycinate: approximately 400 mg for adult men, 320 mg for adult women (apparently this number does not change with the amount of daily D3 or K2).[99]

The ratio in simple terms: If you take 5,000 IU of D3 a day, you would take 50 mcg of K2 a day and about 400 mg of magnesium. If you take 20,000 IU of D3 a day, you would take 200 mcg of K2 a day and about 400 mg of magnesium. If you take 40,000 IU of D3 a day, you would take 400 mcg of K2 a day and about 400 mg of magnesium per day.

(*Important warning*: As there is no concurrence in the medical world concerning RDAs, these figures must be considered arbitrary. Additionally, due to hundreds if not thousands of factors, both known and unknown, you, your

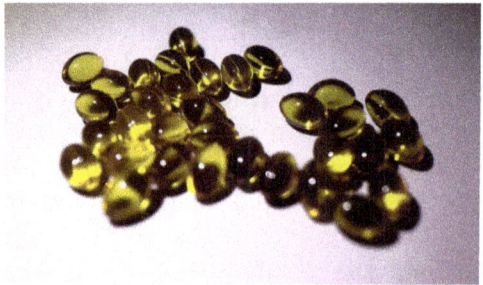

Photograph by Lochlainn Seabrook. Copyright © Lochlainn Seabrook.

body, your nutritional needs, and your health issues are completely unique. Thus, always check with your doctor to determine the correct amount of each vitamin and mineral for your individual situation.)

ONE MUST UTILIZE ALL THREE SOURCES

Having covered the three primary sources of vitamin D3, we must face an uncomfortable reality: In our high-tech day and age we can no longer get enough quality vitamin D3 from the sun alone, from food alone, or from supplements alone.

The solution?

One must try to get their daily dose of vitamin D3 from all three sources whenever possible. This is the best assurance one has for warding off vitamin D deficiencies and the many grievous health hazards that accompany them.

TESTING BLOOD LEVELS

The most accurate method (some say the *only* accurate method) of determining and monitoring your body's current level of vitamin D is to have your blood tested for it. Many mainstream doctors have little knowledge or interest in vitamin D, so you may have to be insistent in requesting this specific test, and also in making sure that it actually measures for vitamin D. If your request fails or if it is not practical, there are a number of do-it-yourself, home vitamin D blood testing kits now available on the market.

Let me point out here that one of the main reasons mainstream medical doctors know so little about D3 is because it is incorrectly considered, and is actually called, a "vitamin," which automatically places it in the field of food science. Unfortunately, orthodox doctors get very little training in food science at medical school.[100] If, however, medical teachers referred to vitamin D by what it actually is—that is, a hormone—it would be considered a *medical* rather than a *nutritional* topic, and it would thus be included in mainstream medical courses on *endocrinology* rather than dismissed as a "medically unrelated" branch of food science, one known as nutrition. Naturally, doctors well-versed on the subject of *hormone* D would be far better equipped to help patients who come to them with problems related to *vitamin* D.[101]

As might be expected, what is considered the "normal" vitamin D blood level varies from country to country, and even from doctor to doctor. Add to this the fact, as noted above, that humans vary considerably from person to person. Nonetheless, generally speaking, a blood test should show a vitamin D level of between 50 ng/dl (that is, nanograms per deciliter) and 80 ng/dl. Anything below 20 ng/dl almost certainly indicates a deficiency, while, according to mainstream medicine, anything above 100 ng/dl to 150 ng/dl is taking you into the toxic (and dangerous) range; though note that some natural doctors consider the latter range "normal."[102]

These numbers suggest that a range of 60-70 ng/dl is optimal, while numbers below or above this may be problematic. Only your doctor's analysis, one that takes into account all of your individual variables, from genetics and lifestyle, to age, diet, skin color, race, and weight, can provide an accurate assessment of what your specific blood numbers mean.

If your numbers are too low, your doctor will probably want to put you on a high therapeutic daily dosage of vitamin D3 for a few days, weeks, or even months, depending on a variety of factors. According to orthodox medicine, one reason knowing and regularly monitoring your blood levels is so important is to avoid overdosing on vitamin D, which, as just mentioned, can lead to a toxic condition known as hypercalcemia—elevated levels of calcium in the blood. In extreme cases this can cause calcification of soft tissue, kidney failure, cardiovascular damage, and even coma.[103]

Other signs of excess vitamin D (or conversely a magnesium and/or vitamin K2 deficiency),[104] are nausea, constipation, anorexia, polyuria, headaches, seizures, high blood pressure, retarded growth, and calcium deposits in the kidneys, heart, and blood vessels.[105] Since, depending on your overall lifestyle—including sun exposure and diet—your body's biochemistry changes from week to week, it is recommended that you get your blood checked for its vitamin D level about every three months (some say every six months). Since this period of time will be different for each individual, always follow the counsel of your doctor.[106]

WHO SHOULD USE EXTRA CAUTION IN TAKING VITAMIN D

Some ailments can pose a risk when combined with high-dose vitamin D therapy. Those with hyperparathyroidism, kidney disease, and sarcoidosis, for example, should work with a certified health practitioner before taking vitamin D supplements. Also, many medications interfere with vitamin D and vice versa, such as cardiac glycosides and thiazide diuretics.[107] Always err on the side of caution by consulting a certified medical professional before embarking on any new dietary regimen.

A WORD ON PETS

Unsurprisingly, anything with a spine, which would include mammals, birds, and reptiles, all possess the same biological need for vitamin D3 that humans do. Proof for this assertion is readily available: We are all familiar with the love our pet cats have for lounging in sunny windows, our pet dogs show for wanting to go outside and play whenever possible, for snakes and lizards sunbathing on exposed rocks, and for the obvious enjoyment birds get from sitting in the sun, often with their wings fanned open (to get as much UVB ray exposure as possible).

These are all methods nonhuman animals use in their attempt to fulfill their daily requirement for vitamin D. Pets that are prevented from getting their daily sun will acquire many of the same ailments that vitamin D deficient humans develop, from, for example, obesity, hair loss, tumors, and cancer, to arthritis, influenza, gingivitis, and depression. Is there a connection? Absolutely, and getting plenty of sunshine is part of the solution.

Consult a knowledgeable veterinarian for other ways to keep your pets vitamin D-healthy—and also to learn how, if needed, to supplement their diet with the proper amount of natural (nontoxic) vitamin D3.[108]

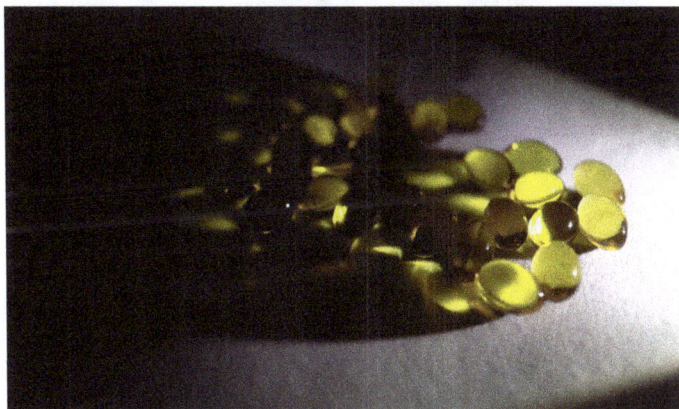

Photograph by Lochlainn Seabrook. Copyright © Lochlainn Seabrook.

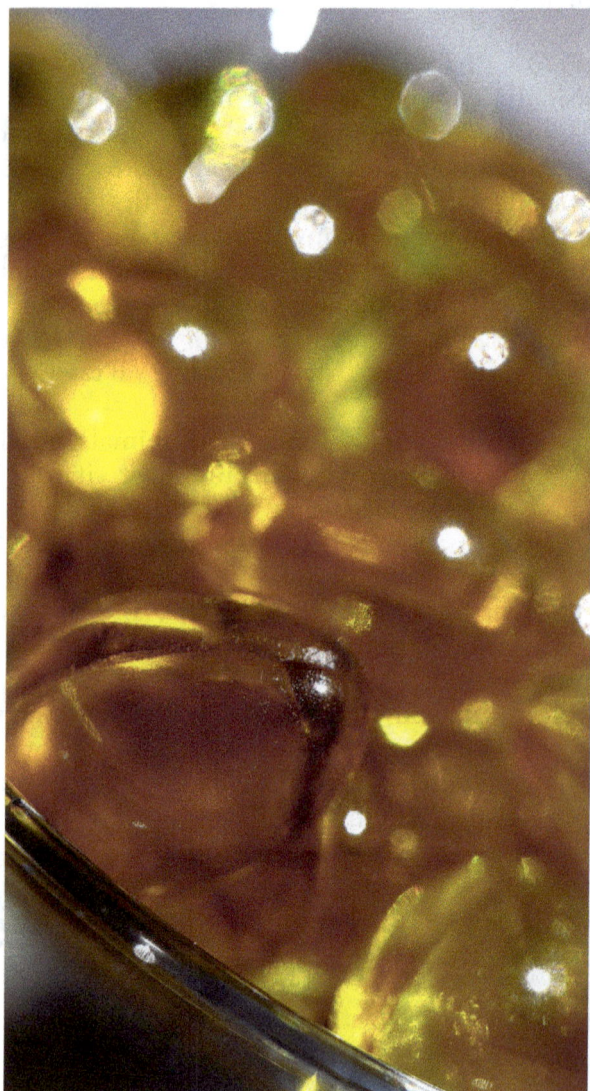

Photograph by Lochlainn Seabrook. Copyright © Lochlainn Seabrook.

CHAPTER 3

SYMPTOMS OF VITAMIN D DEFICIENCY: THE LIST

THE WORLD'S MOST COMMON VITAMIN DEFICIENCY
Naturally, due to the enormous difficulty of getting enough daily vitamin D3, coupled with heliophobia, mainstream medical iatrogenic deceptions, the cosmetic industry's concocted concerns over sun exposure, and the grossly insufficient mainstream RDA, lack of vitamin D is "the most common nutritional deficiency worldwide."[109] It is a pandemic, in fact,[110] with some estimates ranging as high as 97 percent of the global population being vitamin D deficient.[111]

One American study found that "most people in the United States consume less than the recommended amounts of vitamin D"—that is, 600 IU daily—with, alarmingly, the average man getting only around 200 IU a day from foods and women only around 170 IU from foods[112]—far below the alternative medical RDA of 5,000 to 10,000 IU.[113]

Other studies find that in the United Kingdom 90 percent of British adults are vitamin D deficient; 82 percent of the people in India are vitamin D deficient; 82 percent of Japanese people are vitamin D deficient; and 100 percent of the people of Brazil are vitamin D deficient.[114]

THOSE PRONE TO VITAMIN D DEFICIENCY
Who is most apt to being deficient in vitamin D? The elderly, the housebound, the obese, alcoholics, vegans and vegetarians, fruitarians, diabetics, pregnant women, lactating women, postmenopausal women, low income households, those who

eschew dairy and egg products, daylight avoiders, sunlight haters, sunscreen users,[115] those who live in cold high elevations, regions with high air pollution, areas with little daily sunlight,[116] and dark-skinned individuals and races (African-Americans, for example, require as much as 30 times the amount of sunlight to create the same amount of vitamin D in their bodies as European-Americans).[117]

People who are exposed to toxins, as well as those with cystic fibrosis, gout, intestinal diseases, kidney disease, liver disease, thyroid problems, and pancreatic illnesses also have more of a tendency toward vitamin D deficiency than others.[118] (In some cases these ailments are actually *caused* by vitamin D deficiency.)

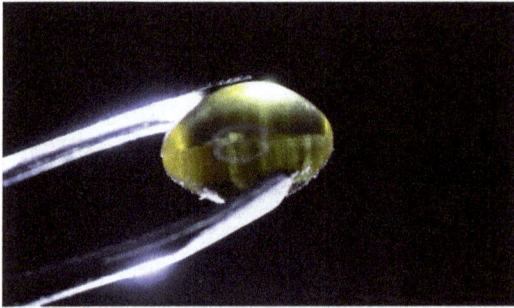

Photograph by Lochlainn Seabrook. Copyright © Lochlainn Seabrook.

According to Dr. Sten Ekberg, "there is virtually no body function where vitamin D is not involved," which is why the vitamin D level, both in your blood and in your cells (these are two separate measures), are excellent biomarkers of overall health.[119] And it is also due to this fact that a deficiency in vitamin D can wreak havoc on the body and on one's life, touching upon nearly every bodily and mental function. It can even cause death, one of the reasons for which it is sometimes called the "silent killer."

As just one example: Researchers at the University of California San Diego School of Medicine found that a vitamin D deficiency can actually cause cancer, for "higher levels of vitamin D are associated with a correspondingly reduced risk of cancer."[120] In fact, currently vitamin D has been found to be related to risk reduction in at least 17 different forms of cancer.[121] Personally, I have no doubt that eventually all 200 cancer subtypes will be linked to vitamin D in some way.[122]

LIST OF SYMPTOMS OF VITAMIN D DEFICIENCY
Now that we have covered the definition, functions, RDA, and sources of vitamin D, it is time to look at the many symptoms of vitamin D deficiency, the most convenient way which is in registry form. I spent many months researching, preparing, and compiling the following list for this book—making it the only work of its kind.

This massive record is invaluable as it should be able to help you pinpoint the direction you may need to go in as far as medical advice and vitamin D therapy. Although occasionally some D deficient individuals may show no symptoms (that is, they are asymptomatic), in general the average sufferer will present one or more of the conditions I have listed below.

HOW TO USE THE LIST
To use this alphabetical list, look up the name (common or medical) of the specific disease or ailment you are interested in and go to its endnote at the back of the book; from there read the appended information or article(s)—sources I have attached to assist you in furthering your own research. I am not a doctor, scientist, or nutritionist. I cannot vouch for the truth, validity, accuracy, or pertinence of this material. It is up to you and your physician to determine if and how they apply to you.

IMPORTANT NOTES
◆ I have listed some conditions by more than one name.
◆ Some ailments have additional names, both scientific and colloquial, that I have not listed here.
◆ By some estimates there are at least 26,000 human diseases.[123] My list of 1,000 or so of the most commonly known diseases represents only a small fraction of these—a little less than 4 percent of the total. Thus, if your ailment is not listed here, it does not mean that it is not associated with vitamin D in some way. It almost certainly is, as the vast majority of human illnesses are vitamin D-related.
◆ For the purposes of both impartiality and supplying well-rounded information, in some cases I have appended anti-vitamin D therapy information, studies, and articles, or material that is only distantly related to vitamin D.

◆ As noted, the information and articles I have selected may or may not be applicable to your particular health situation, or, in some cases, even to vitamin D specifically. However, I have tried to select information connected to vitamin D in some way, even if remotely or indirectly.

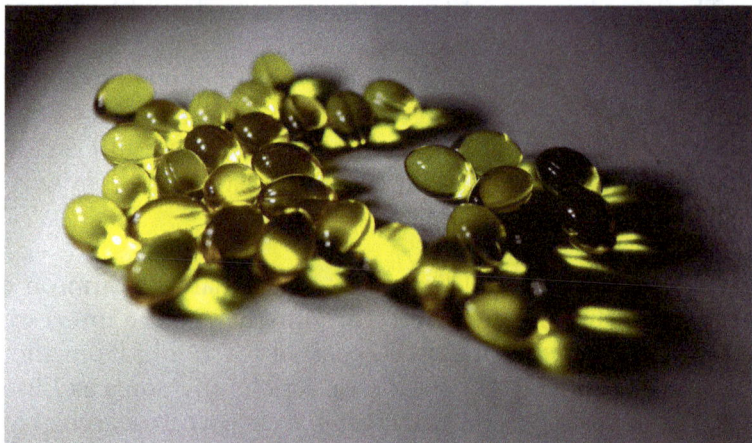

Photograph by Lochlainn Seabrook. Copyright © Lochlainn Seabrook.

◆ Show your doctor this book, and discuss your questions and concerns with them. Hopefully he or she will be receptive. Amazingly, but perhaps not surprisingly, many conventional doctors and medical/scientific organizations do not believe that vitamin D has any direct association with disease. The thousands of vitamin D-related papers, studies, and research I cite in my endnotes (some of them going back nearly 100 years), along with my own many vitamin D-related healings, completely refute this view, however.

◆ Your health is never static. It is always dynamic. The body is constantly remodeling itself,[124] repairing cells, creating new tissues, rebuilding bones, etc.[125] Because of this, the conditions itemized in this list will manifest differently in different people and at different times in their lives—yet another important reason to *always* seek the advice, help, and care of a licensed physician when dealing with your health.

THE LIST OF
HYPOVITAMINOSIS D-RELATED AILMENTS
Over 1,000 Disorders & Diseases Caused by Vitamin D Deficiency
(or in some cases conditions that are preventable or treatable using vitamin D)

AAA (abdominal aortic aneurysm).[126]
Abdominal aortic aneurysm (AAA).[127]
Abdominal pain.[128]
Abetalipoproteinemia.[129]
Achromatopsia.[130]
Acne.[131]
Acquired immunodeficiency syndrome (AIDS).[132]
Acromegaly.[133]
Actinic keratosis.[134]
Acute coronary syndrome.[135]
Acute intermittent porphyria.[136]
Acute pancreatitis.[137]
Acute respiratory distress syndrome (ARDS).[138]
Addictions.[139]
Addictive personality disorder.[140]
Addison's disease.[141]
Adenitis.[142]
Adenomyosis.[143]
ADHD (attention-deficit/hyperactivity disorder).[144]
Adhesive capsulitis (frozen shoulder).[145]
Adrenoleukodystrophy.[146]
Adult T-cell leukemia/lymphoma (ATL).[147]
Advanced sleep phase disorder.[148]
AGAT deficiency.[149]
Age-related macular degeneration.[150]
Aging, premature.[151]
Agoraphobia.[152]
Agnosia.[153]
AIDS (acquired immunodeficiency syndrome).[154]
Alagille syndrome.[155]
Alcoholism.[156]
Alkaptonuria.[157]
Allergic diseases.[158]
Allergic rhinitis (hay fever).[159]
Alopecia areata.[160]

ALS (Amyotrophic lateral sclerosis, or Lou Gehrig's disease).[161]
Alzheimer's disease.[162]
Amnesia.[163]
Amphetamines dependence.[164]
Amyloidosis.[165]
Amyotrophic lateral sclerosis (ALS, or Lou Gehrig's disease).[166]
Anaphylaxis.[167]
Androgen insensitivity syndrome.[168]
Anemia (iron deficiency).[169]
Anger.[170]
Angina.[171]
Angioedema.[172]
Ankles, clicking, popping, or cracking.[173]
Ankles, easily sprained.[174]
Ankylosing spondylitis.[175]
Anorexia nervosa.[176]
Antiphospholipid syndrome (APS).[177]
Antisocial personality disorder (APD).[178]
Anxiety.[179]
Aortic aneurysm.[180]
Aphthous stomatitis.[181]
Appendicitis.[182]
Appetite, reduced or loss of.[183]
APS (antiphospholipid syndrome).[184]
ARDS (acute respiratory distress syndrome).[185]
Arrhythmogenic right ventricular dysplasia.[186]
Arterial disease.[187]
Arterial thrombosis.[188]
Arthritis.[189]
Atrial fibrillation.[190]
ASD (autistic spectrum disorder).[191]
Asperger's syndrome.[192]
Aspergillosis.[193]
Asthma.[194]
Ataxia.[195]
Atherosclerosis.[196]
Athletes' foot.[197]
Athletic performance.[198]

Atopic dermatitis.[199]
Atopic eczema.[200]
Atrial fibrillation.[201]
Atrial heart septal defect.[202]
Attention-deficit disorder (ADD).[203]
Attention-deficit/hyperactivity disorder (ADHD).[204]
Autism.[205]
Autistic spectrum disorder (ASD).[206]
Auto brewery syndrome.[207]
Autoimmune-inflammatory diseases.[208]
Autoimmune thyroiditis.[209]
Babesiosis.[210]
Back pain (lower).[211]
Bacterial infections.[212]
Bacterial vaginosis.[213]
Barakat syndrome or HDR syndrome (hypoparathyroidism,
    sensorineural deafness, and renal disease).[214]
Basal cell nevus syndrome (BCNS).[215]
Bazex-Dupré-Christol syndrome.[216]
BDD (body dysmorphic disorder).[217]
Behavior.[218]
Behcet's disease.[219]
Benign mesothelioma.[220]
Benign paroxysmal positional vertigo (BPPV).[221]
Benign prostate enlargement.[222]
Bent bones.[223]
Berardinelli-Seip congenital lipodystrophy.[224]
Bile duct cancer (cholangiocarcinoma).[225]
Binge eating.[226]
Bipolar disorder.[227]
Bladder cancer.[228]
Bladder infections.[229]
Blindness.[230]
Blocked arteries (coronary heart disease).[231]
Blood cancers.[232]
Blood clotting (thrombosis).[233]
Blount disease.[234]
BMS (burning mouth syndrome).[235]
Body aches and pain.[236]
Body dysmorphic disorder (BDD).[237]

Body integrity dysphoria (BID).[238]
Bone cancer.[239]
Bone chips.[240]
Bone deformities.[241]
Bone disease.[242]
Bone fractures.[243]
Bone health.[244]
Bone loss.[245]
Bone pain.[246]
Bone spurs.[247]
Bone weakness.[248]
Borderline personality disorder.[249]
Bowed legs.[250]
Bowel cancer.[251]
Bowel incontinence.[252]
Bowel polyps.[253]
BPPV (benign paroxysmal positional vertigo).[254]
Brain aneurysm (intracranial aneurysm).[255]
Brain deformities (children).[256]
Brain lesions.[257]
Brain stem death.[258]
Brain tumors.[259]
Breast cancer.[260]
Broken bones, history of.[261]
Bronchiectasis.[262]
Bronchitis.[263]
Bronchopulmonary dysplasia.[264]
Brooke-Spiegler syndrome.[265]
Brucellosis.[266]
Brugada syndrome.[267]
Bruxism.[268]
Buck teeth (overbite).[269]
Bulimia.[270]
Bullying (and being bullied).[271]
Bunions (hallux valgus).[272]
Burning mouth syndrome (BMS).[273]
Burns.[274]
CAD (coronary artery disease).[275]
Caffeine dependence (coffee).[276]
Calciphylaxis.[277]

Canavan disease.[278]
Candida albicans.[279]
Candidiasis infections.[280]
Canker sores.[281]
Carcinoid syndrome.[282]
Carcinoid tumors.[283]
Cardiovascular disease (CVD).[284]
Carpal tunnel syndrome.[285]
Cataplexy.[286]
Cataracts.[287]
Catatonia.[288]
Catecholaminergic polymorphic ventricular tachycardia.[289]
Celiac (or coeliac) disease.[290]
Cerebral palsy.[291]
Cerebrovascular accident (stroke).[292]
Cervical adenitis.[293]
Cervical cancer.[294]
Cervical spondylosis.[295]
Cesarean section.[296]
CFS (chronic fatigue syndrome).[297]
Chapped lips (cheilitis).[298]
Cheilitis (chapped lips).[299]
Chest illnesses.[300]
Chest infection.[301]
Chest pain (angina).[302]
Chickenpox (varicella zoster virus).[303]
Chilblains.[304]
Chlamydia trachomatis.[305]
Cholangiocarcinoma (bile duct cancer).[306]
Cholangitis.[307]
Cholera (vibrio cholerae).[308]
Chorioamnionitis.[309]
Chorioretinopathy.[310]
Chronic coronary syndrome.[311]
Chronic fatigue syndrome (CFS) or myalgic encephalomyelitis (ME).[312]
Chronic lymphocytic leukaemia.[313]
Chronic myeloid leukaemia.[314]
Chronic obstructive pulmonary disease (COPD).[315]
Chronic pain.[316]

Chronic pancreatitis.[317]
Circadian rhythm sleep disorder.[318]
Cirrhosis.[319]
Citrullinemia.[320]
Clicking bones.[321]
Cluster headaches.[322]
Clostridium difficile.[323]
Cocaine dependence.[324]
Cochlear otosclerosis.[325]
Coeliac (or celiac) disease.[326]
Coffee dependence (caffeine).[327]
Cognitive function, reduced.[328]
Cold sores.[329]
Colitis.[330]
Colon cancer.[331]
Colorectal cancer.[332]
Coma.[333]
Common cold.[334]
Complex regional pain syndrome.[335]
Complex post-traumatic stress disorder (CPTSD).[336]
Compulsive sexual behavior disorder (sex addiction).[337]
Concentration, lack of.[338]
Conduct disorder.[339]
Condyloma acuminata (genital warts).[340]
Confusion.[341]
Confusional arousals.[342]
Congenital heart block.[343]
Congenital heart disease.[344]
Congenital hyperinsulinism.[345]
Congenital ichthyosis.[346]
Conjunctivitis.[347]
Connective tissue disease.[348]
Constipation.[349]
Convulsions.[350]
COPD (chronic obstructive pulmonary disease).[351]
Coronary artery disease (CAD).[352]
Coronary heart disease.[353]
Coronary syndrome.[354]
Coronavirus (COVID-19).[355]
Costello syndrome.[356]

Costochondritis.[357]
Cough.[358]
COVID-19 (coronavirus).[359]
Cowden syndrome.[360]
CPTSD (complex post-traumatic stress disorder).[361]
Craniosynostosis.[362]
Crohn's disease.[363]
Croup.[364]
Cushing's syndrome.[365]
Cutis laxa.[366]
CVD (cardiovascular disease).[367]
Cystic fibrosis.[368]
Cystitis.[369]
Cysts.[370]
Dandruff.[371]
Deafness.[372]
Deep vein thrombosis.[373]
Degenerative cervical myelopathy.[374]
Deletion syndrome.[375]
Delayed sleep phase disorder.[376]
Delirium.[377]
Delusional disorder.[378]
Dementia.[379]
Dental abscess.[380]
Dental agenesis.[381]
Dental diseases.[382]
Denys-Drash syndrome.[383]
Depression.[384]
Dermatitis.[385]
Dermatitis herpetiformis (Duhring's disease).[386]
Despair.[387]
Developmental delay in children.[388]
Developmental dysplasia.[389]
Diabetes 1 and 2.[390]
Diabetic peripheral neuropathy (DPN).[391]
Diabetic retinopathy.[392]
Diarrhea.[393]
Diamond-Blackfan anemia.[394]
Digestive disorders.[395]
DiGeorge syndrome.[396]

Digital addiction.[397]
Diphtheria.[398]
Disc herniation (herniated disc).[399]
Discoid eczema.[400]
Disruptive mood dysregulation disorder.[401]
Disseminated intravascular coagulation.[402]
Distal arthrogryposis.[403]
Diverticular disease.[404]
Diverticulitis.[405]
Dizziness.[406]
Down syndrome.[407]
DPN (diabetic peripheral neuropathy).[408]
Dreams.[409]
Dry eye syndrome.[410]
Duhring's disease (dermatitis herpetiformis).[411]
Dysgeusia.[412]
Dyslexia.[413]
Dyspepsia.[414]
Dysphagia.[415]
Dysthymia.[416]
Dystonia.[417]
Earache (and infections).[418]
Eating, difficulty.[419]
Eating disorders.[420]
Ebola virus disease.[421]
Ectopic pregnancy.[422]
Eczema.[423]
EDS (Ehlers-Danlos syndrome).[424]
Edwards' syndrome.[425]
Ehlers-Danlos syndrome (EDS).[426]
Ehrlichiosis.[427]
Emphysema.[428]
Endogenous alcohol fermentation syndrome.[429]
Endometrial Cancer.[430]
Endometriosis.[431]
Endurance, reduced.[432]
Energy, loss of.[433]
Enlarged vestibular aqueduct syndrome (EVAS).[434]
Enuresis.[435]
Eosinophilic esophagitis.[436]

EPI (exocrine pancreatic insufficiency).[437]
Epilepsy.[438]
Epistaxis (nose bleed).[439]
Epstein-Barr virus.[440]
Erectile dysfunction (in men).[441]
Erythema infectiosum (slapped cheek syndrome).[442]
Erythropoietic protoporphyria.[443]
Escherichia coli.[444]
Esophageal atresia.[445]
Esophageal varices.[446]
Essential hypernatremia syndrome.[447]
Ewing sarcoma (peripheral primitive neuroectodermal tumor).[448]
Excoriation disorder (skin picking disorder).[449]
Eye cancer.[450]
Eye issues.[451]
Exocrine pancreatic insufficiency (EPI).[452]
Factor VII deficiency.[453]
Fahr's syndrome (or disease).[454]
Falls (falling).[455]
Familial adenomatous polyposis.[456]
Familial combined hyperlipidemia.[457]
Familial chylomicronemia syndrome.[458]
Fanconi anemia.[459]
Farsightedness (hyperopia).[460]
Fatigue.[461]
Fatty tumors (lipoma).[462]
Febrile seizures.[463]
Fecal incontinence.[464]
Female specific conditions.[465]
Fetal alcohol syndrome.[466]
Fever.[467]
Fibrodysplasia ossificans progressiva.[468]
Fibroids.[469]
Fibromyalgia.[470]
Fingernail fungus.[471]
Flu.[472]
FND (functional neurological disorder).[473]
Focus, inability to.[474]
Forgetfulness.[475]

Food addiction.[476]
Food allergies.[477]
Foot fungus.[478]
Foot issues.[479]
Foot ulcers.[480]
Frequent illnesses.[481]
Frozen shoulder (adhesive capsulitis).[482]
Functional dyspepsia.[483]
Functional gastrointestinal disorders (FGS).[484]
Functional neurological disorder (FND).[485]
Fungal infections.[486]
Fungal nail infection.[487]
G6PD deficiency (glucose-6-phosphate dehydrogenase deficiency).[488]
Galactosemia.[489]
Gallbladder cancer.[490]
Gallstones.[491]
Ganglion cysts.[492]
Gangliosidoses.[493]
Gastritis.[494]
Gastroesophageal reflux disease (GERD).[495]
Gastroenteritis.[496]
Gastrointestinal disease.[497]
Gastrointestinal stromal tumor.[498]
Gastro-oesophageal reflux disease (GORD).[499]
Gaucher Disease.[500]
GCA (Horton's disease or giant cell arteritis).[501]
Gender dysphoria.[502]
Generalized anxiety disorder.[503]
Genetic aging.[504]
Genital warts (condyloma acuminata).[505]
Genitourinary syndrome.[506]
GERD (gastroesophageal reflux disease).[507]
Germ cell tumours.[508]
Gestational diabetes.[509]
Gestational trophoblastic neoplasm.[510]
Getting sick easily and frequently.[511]
GI (gastrointestinal issues).[512]
Giant cell arteritis or Horton's disease (GCA).[513]
Giardiasis.[514]

Gingivitis.[515]
Glandular fever.[516]
Glanzmann thrombasthenia.[517]
Glaucoma.[518]
Glucose-6-phosphate dehydrogenase deficiency (G6PD deficiency).[519]
Glycogen storage disease.[520]
Golfer's elbow (medial epicondylitis).[521]
Gonorrhea.[522]
GORD (gastro-oesophageal reflux disease).[523]
Gorlin-Goltz syndrome.[524]
Gout.[525]
Graves' Disease.[526]
Greater trochanteric pain syndrome.[527]
Grover's disease.[528]
Growing pains.[529]
Grumpiness.[530]
Guillain-Barré syndrome.[531]
Gum disease.[532]
Gum inflammation.[533]
Gums, bleeding.[534]
Gut fermentation syndrome.[535]
Guttate psoriasis.[536]
H1N1 (including influenza).[537]
Hair growth, slowing of.[538]
Hair loss/thinning.[539]
Hallucinations.[540]
Hallux valgus (bunions).[541]
Hand, foot and mouth disease.[542]
Hardening of the arteries (atherosclerosis).[543]
Hashimoto's disease.[544]
Hay fever (allergic rhinitis).[545]
HDR syndrome or Barakat syndrome (hypoparathyroidism, sensorineural deafness, and renal disease).[546]
Headaches (often manifesting as pressure on one side).[547]
Head and neck cancer.[548]
Hearing loss.[549]
Heart arrhythmia.[550]
Heart attack.[551]
Heart block.[552]

Heart disease.[553]
Heart failure.[554]
Heart hypertrophy.[555]
Heart palpitations.[556]
Hemophilia.[557]
Hemorrhoids (piles).[558]
Hepatitis.[559]
Hepatitis A.[560]
Hepatitis B.[561]
Hepatitis C.[562]
Hereditary fructose intolerance.[563]
Hereditary spherocytosis.[564]
Hernia (reducible inguinal).[565]
Herniated disc (disc herniation).[566]
Herpes labialis (oral).[567]
Herpes simplex virus (genital).[568]
Herpes zoster (shingles).[569]
High blood pressure (hypertension).[570]
High cholesterol.[571]
Hip-spine syndrome.[572]
Hirschsprung's disease.[573]
Hives (urticaria).[574]
HIV (human immunodeficiency virus).[575]
Hoarding disorder (syllogomania).[576]
Hodgkin's lymphoma.[577]
Homocystinuria.[578]
Hopelessness.[579]
Hormonal changes.[580]
Horton's disease or giant cell arteritis (GCA).[581]
Horton's syndrome.[582]
Human herpesvirus 3 (chickenpox).[583]
Human immunodeficiency virus (HIV).[584]
Hungry bone syndrome.[585]
Huntington's disease.[586]
Hurler's syndrome.[587]
Hyperaldosteronism.[588]
Hyperemesis gravidarum.[589]
Hyperglycemia (high blood sugar).[590]
Hyperhidrosis.[591]
Hyper IgE syndrome.[592]

Hyperopia (farsightedness).[593]
Hyperparathyroidism.[594]
Hyperprolactinemia.[595]
Hyperpyretic syndrome.[596]
Hypersomnia.[597]
Hypertension (high blood pressure).[598]
Hyperthyroidism.[599]
Hypnagogic hallucinations.[600]
Hypobetalipoproteinemia.[601]
Hypoglycemia (low blood sugar).[602]
Hypogonadism.[603]
Hypoparathyroidism.[604]
Hypophosphatemia.[605]
Hypopituitarism.[606]
Hypotension (low blood pressure).[607]
Hypothyroidism.[608]
Hypoxia.[609]
IBD (inflammatory bowel disease).[610]
IBS (irritable bowel syndrome).[611]
Idiopathic nephrotic syndrome.[612]
Idiopathic pulmonary fibrosis.[613]
Idiopathic ventricular fibrillation.[614]
IM (infectious mononucleosis).[615]
Immunity, decreased.[616]
Immune system, weakening of.[617]
Impaired wound healing.[618]
Impetigo herpetiformis.[619]
Incontinence.[620]
Indigestion.[621]
Infections.[622]
Infectious mononucleosis (IM).[623]
Infertility (female).[624]
Infertility (male).[625]
Inflammation.[626]
Inflammatory bowel disease (IBD).[627]
Inflammatory heart diseases.[628]
Influenza (including H1N1).[629]
Immigration (immigrants).[630]
Immune reconstitution inflammatory syndrome.[631]
Inner ear infection (otitis interna).[632]

Insulin resistance.[633]
Insomnia.[634]
Interest, loss of.[635]
Intermittent explosive disorder (IED).[636]
Internet addiction.[637]
Interstitial nephritis.[638]
Intracranial aneurysm (brain aneurysm).[639]
Intrahepatic cholestasis.[640]
Iron deficiency (anemia).[641]
Irregular sleep-wake rhythm.[642]
Irritable bowel syndrome (IBS).[643]
Irritability.[644]
Isolation, by individual.[645]
Itching.[646]
Jaw muscles, loose or weak.[647]
Jet lag.[648]
Jeune syndrome.[649]
Joints, deformities in.[650]
Joint hypermobility.[651]
Joint infections.[652]
Joint pain.[653]
Kallmann syndrome.[654]
Kaposi's sarcoma.[655]
Kasabach-Meritt syndrome.[656]
Kawasaki disease.[657]
Kearns-Sayre syndrome.[658]
Keratoconjunctivitis.[659]
Kidney cancer.[660]
Kidney disease.[661]
Kidney infections.[662]
Kidney stones.[663]
Klebsiella pneumoniae.[664]
Knee diseases.[665]
Knee pain.[666]
Knuckles, cracking.[667]
Kwashiorkor syndrome.[668]
Labyrinthitis.[669]
Lactating women.[670]
Lactose intolerance.[671]
Laryngeal (larynx) cancer.[672]

Laryngeal dystonia (spasmodic dysphonia).[673]
Laryngitis.[674]
Lateral epicondylitis (tennis elbow).[675]
Learning disabilities (adults).[676]
Learning disabilities (children).[677]
Leg cramps.[678]
Legionnaires' disease.[679]
Leukemia.[680]
Leukodystrophy.[681]
Leukopenia.[682]
Libido.[683]
Lichen planus.[684]
Ligament pain.[685]
Lipid issues.[686]
Lipoedema.[687]
Lipoma (fatty tumor).[688]
Liver cancer.[689]
Liver disease.[690]
Liver tumors.[691]
Loeys-Dietz syndrome.[692]
Long QT syndrome.[693]
Loss of appetite.[694]
Lou Gehrig's disease.[695]
Lower back pain (lumbago).[696]
Lumbar stenosis.[697]
Lung cancer.[698]
Lung injuries.[699]
Lung issues.[700]
Lupus (systemic lupus erythematosus or SLE).[701]
Lyme disease.[702]
Lymphoedema.[703]
Lymphogranuloma venereum.[704]
Lymphoma.[705]
Lynch syndrome.[706]
Macular degeneration.[707]
MAFLD (metabolic dysfunction-associated fatty liver disease).[708]
Mahaim syndrome.[709]
Major depressive disorder.[710]
Malabsorption syndrome.[711]

Malaria.[712]
Malignant growths.[713]
Malignant pleural mesothelioma.[714]
Malocclusion (dental defects).[715]
Manic depression.[716]
Maple syrup urine disease.[717]
Marfan syndrome.[718]
MCTD (mixed connective tissue disease).[719]
Measles.[720]
Medial epicondylitis (golfer's elbow).[721]
Medications.[722]
Mediterranean fever.[723]
Melancholy.[724]
Melanoma (skin cancer).[725]
Memory loss.[726]
Meniere's disease.[727]
Meningitis.[728]
Meningoencephalitis.[729]
Mental disorders.[730]
Mental health.[731]
Menopause.[732]
Menstrual cramps.[733]
Mesothelioma.[734]
Metabolic dysfunction-associated fatty liver disease (MAFLD).[735]
Metabolic syndrome.[736]
Methylmalonic acidemia.[737]
Mevalonic aciduria.[738]
Mixed connective tissue disease (MCTD).[739]
Muenke syndrome.[740]
Middle ear infection (otitis media).[741]
Migraine headaches.[742]
Milkman's syndrome.[743]
Miscarriage.[744]
MND (motor neurone disease).[745]
Mood changes.[746]
Mood disorders.[747]
Mood swings.[748]
Morgagni syndrome.[749]
Motor neurone disease (MND).[750]

Mouth cancer.[751]
Mouth ulcers.[752]
MS (multiple sclerosis).[753]
MSA (multiple system atrophy).[754]
Multiple myeloma.[755]
Multiple sclerosis (MS).[756]
Multiple system atrophy (MSA).[757]
Mumps (parotitis).[758]
Munchausen's syndrome.[759]
Muscle aches.[760]
Muscle cramps.[761]
Muscle loss (sarcopenia).[762]
Muscle twitches.[763]
Muscle weakness.[764]
Musculoskeletal pain.[765]
Myalgic encephalomyelitis (ME) or chronic fatigue syndrome
   (CFS).[766]
Myasthenia gravis.[767]
Myocardial infarction.[768]
Myopia (nearsightedness).[769]
Myositis ossificans progressiva.[770]
Myotonic dystrophy.[771]
NAFLD (non-alcoholic fatty liver disease).[772]
Narcissism.[773]
Narcissistic personality disorder.[774]
Narcolepsy.[775]
Nasal and sinus cancer.[776]
NASH (non-alcoholic steatohepatitis).[777]
Nearsightedness (myopia).[778]
Neck pain.[779]
Nephrogenic diabetes insipidus.[780]
Nephrolithiasis (kidney stones).[781]
Nervousness.[782]
Nervous system diseases.[783]
Neurilemmoma.[784]
Neuroblastoma.[785]
Neurofibromatosis.[786]
Neurohypophyseal diabetes insipidus.[787]
Neuropathy.[788]
Neuropsychiatric disease.[789]

Neuropsychiatric lupus.[790]
Neuroticism.[791]
Neutropenia.[792]
Nevoid hyperkeratosis.[793]
Newborns, underweight.[794]
NHL (non-Hodgkin's lymphoma).[795]
Nicotine (smoking).[796]
Night eating syndrome.[797]
Nightmares.[798]
Night terrors (sleep terrors).[799]
Non-alcoholic fatty liver disease (NAFLD).[800]
Non-alcoholic steatohepatitis (NASH).[801]
Non-Hodgkin's lymphoma (NHL).[802]
Non-melanoma skin cancer.[803]
Noonan syndrome (NS).[804]
Norovirus.[805]
Nose bleed (epistaxis).[806]
NS (Noonan syndrome).[807]
Numbness.[808]
Obesity.[809]
Obsessive compulsive disorder (OCD).[810]
Obstructive sleep apnea.[811]
OCD (obsessive compulsive disorder).[812]
Ocular diseases.[813]
Oesophageal cancer.[814]
Olfactory reference syndrome.[815]
Opioid dependence.[816]
Oppositional defiant disorder.[817]
Oral lichen planus.[818]
Oral cavity diseases.[819]
Oral mucositis.[820]
Oral thrush.[821]
Osteoarthritis.[822]
Osteochondrodysplasias.[823]
Osteogenesis imperfecta.[824]
Osteomalacia (adult rickets).[825]
Osteopenia.[826]
Osteoporosis.[827]
Osteosarcoma.[828]
Otitis interna (inner ear infection).[829]

Otitis media (middle ear infection).[830]
Otitis externa (outer ear infection).[831]
Otosclerosis.[832]
Outer ear infection (otitis externa).[833]
Ovarian cancer.[834]
Ovarian cyst.[835]
Overactive thyroid.[836]
Paget's disease.[837]
Pain, chronic widespread.[838]
Pain, increased sensitivity to.[839]
Pale skin.[840]
Pancreatic cancer.[841]
Pancreatitis.[842]
Panic disorder (attacks).[843]
Paraganglioma.[844]
Paralysis.[845]
Paraneoplastic syndrome.[846]
Paranoid personality disorder.[847]
Paraphrenia.[848]
Parasites.[849]
Parathyroid adenoma.[850]
Parkinson's disease.[851]
Parotitis (mumps).[852]
Passive-aggressive personality disorder.[853]
Patellofemoral pain syndrome.[854]
PCOS (polycystic ovary syndrome).[855]
PCP (pneumocystis pneumonia).[856]
Pearson's syndrome.[857]
Pediatric inflammatory multisystem syndrome (PIMS).[858]
Pelvic inflammatory disease.[859]
Pelvic organ prolapse.[860]
Pendred syndrome.[861]
Penile cancer.[862]
Peptic ulcer.[863]
Periodic fever.[864]
Periodontal gum disease.[865]
Periodontitis.[866]
Periorbital hyperpigmentation (POH).[867]
Peripheral arterial disease.[868]
Peripheral neuropathy (PN).[869]

Peripheral primitive neuroectodermal tumor (Ewing sarcoma).[870]
Pernicious anemia.[871]
Peroxisomal disorders.[872]
Personality disorder.[873]
Pesticides, exposure to.[874]
Peutz-Jeghers syndrome.[875]
PFAPA syndrome (periodic fevers, with aphthous stomatitis, pharyngitis, and adenitis).[876]
Pharyngitis.[877]
Phenylketonuria.[878]
Phlebitis (vein inflammation).[879]
Photosensitivity (skin light sensitivity).[880]
Pica.[881]
Piles (hemorrhoids).[882]
Pilomatricoma.[883]
PIMS (pediatric inflammatory multisystem syndrome).[884]
Pituitary adenoma (benign tumor).[885]
Pituitary tumor.[886]
Pityriasis rosea.[887]
Pityriasis rubra pilaris (PRB).[888]
Plantar fasciitis.[889]
Plantar heel pain.[890]
Plantar warts.[891]
Pleurisy.[892]
Plummer-Vinson syndrome (PVS).[893]
PMS (pre-menstrual symptoms).[894]
PN (peripheral neuropathy).[895]
Pneumocystis pneumonia (PCP).[896]
Pneumonia.[897]
POH (periorbital hyperpigmentation).[898]
Polio.[899]
Poliomyelitis.[900]
Polycythemia vera.[901]
Polycystic kidney disease.[902]
Polycystic liver disease.[903]
Polycystic ovary syndrome (PCOS).[904]
Polymyalgia rheumatica.[905]
Postmenopausal osteoporosis.[906]
Postpartum depression.[907]

Post traumatic stress disorder (PTSD).[908]
Postural orthostatic tachycardia syndrome (POTS).[909]
POTS (postural orthostatic tachycardia syndrome).[910]
Prader-Willi syndrome.[911]
PRB (pityriasis rubra pilaris).[912]
Preeclampsia.[913]
Pregnancy and newborn issues.[914]
Premature death.[915]
Premenstrual dysphoric disorder.[916]
Premenstrual symptoms (PMS).[917]
Pressure ulcers.[918]
Preterm births.[919]
Primary hyperoxaluria.[920]
Productivity, low.[921]
Progressive supranuclear palsy (PSP).[922]
Propionic acidemia.[923]
Prostate cancer.[924]
Prostate issues.[925]
Proteinuria.[926]
Protein S deficiency.[927]
Pseudohypoaldosteronism.[928]
Pseudohypoparathyroidism.[929]
Psoriasis.[930]
Psoriasis vulgaris.[931]
Psoriatic arthritis.[932]
PSP (progressive supranuclear palsy).[933]
Psychiatric distress.[934]
Psychiatric illnesses.[935]
Psychiatric inpatients.[936]
Psychiatric symptoms.[937]
Psychogenic non-epileptic seizures.[938]
Psychological disorders.[939]
Psychosis.[940]
PTSD (post traumatic stress disorder).[941]
Pulmonary disease.[942]
Pulmonary embolism.[943]
Pulmonary fibrosis.[944]
Pulmonary hypertension.[945]
Purging disorder.[946]
PVS (Plummer-Vinson syndrome).[947]

Pyruvate carboxylase deficiency.[948]
Rapid eye movement sleep behavior disorder.[949]
Rapunzel syndrome (trichobezoar syndrome).[950]
Raynaud's phenomenon.[951]
Reactive arthritis.[952]
Reactive attachment disorder.[953]
Rectus-adductor syndrome.[954]
Recurring infections.[955]
Reflex sympathetic dystrophy syndrome.[956]
Renal failure.[957]
Renal osteodystrophy.[958]
Respiratory infections and illnesses.[959]
Restless legs syndrome.[960]
Retinoblastoma.[961]
Retinopathy.[962]
Rhabdomyosarcoma.[963]
Rheumatoid arthritis.[964]
Rib injuries.[965]
Rickets (childhood).[966]
Ringworm (tinea capitis).[967]
RMSF (Rocky Mountain spotted fever).[968]
Rocky Mountain spotted fever (RMSF).[969]
Rosacea.[970]
Rotator cuff, torn.[971]
RSH-syndrome (Smith-Lemli-Opitz-syndrome).[972]
Rumination syndrome.[973]
SAD (seasonal affective disorder).[974]
Sadness.[975]
Salmonella colitis.[976]
Sarcoidosis.[977]
Sarcopenia (muscle loss).[978]
Saethre-Chotzen syndrome.[979]
SARS (severe acute respiratory syndrome).[980]
Satoyoshi syndrome.[981]
Scabies.[982]
Scarlet fever.[983]
Schizophrenia (childhood and adult).[984]
Schizoid personality disorder.[985]
Sciatica.[986]
Scleroderma (systemic sclerosis).[987]

Scoliosis.[988]
Seasonal affective disorder (SAD).[989]
Seasonal allergic conjunctivitis.[990]
Sex addiction (compulsive sexual behavior disorder, CSBD).[991]
Seborrhoeic keratosis.[992]
Selective mutism.[993]
Self-harm.[994]
Sensitivity to pain, increased.[995]
Sensorineural deafness.[996]
Sepsis.[997]
Septic shock.[998]
Severe acute respiratory syndrome (SARS).[999]
Shared delusional disorder.[1000]
Shingles (herpes zoster).[1001]
Short bowel syndrome.[1002]
Short QT syndrome.[1003]
Shortness of breath.[1004]
SIADH (syndrome of inappropriate antidiuretic hormone).[1005]
Sickle cell anemia.[1006]
Sickle cell disease.[1007]
Sick sinus syndrome.[1008]
Sideroblastic anemia.[1009]
SIDS (sudden infant death syndrome).[1010]
Sinusitis.[1011]
Sjögren syndrome.[1012]
Skin cancer (melanoma).[1013]
Skin cancer (non-melanoma).[1014]
Skin conditions.[1015]
Skin infections.[1016]
Skin light sensitivity (photosensitivity).[1017]
Skin picking disorder (excoriation disorder).[1018]
Skin tags.[1019]
Slapped cheek syndrome (erythema infectiosum).[1020]
SLE (systemic lupus erythematosus).[1021]
Sleep apnea.[1022]
Sleep issues.[1023]
Sleep, poor quality.[1024]
Sleep terrors (night terrors).[1025]
Sleepwalking.[1026]
Smallpox.[1027]

Smell impairment.[1028]
Smith-Lemli-Opitz-syndrome (RSH-syndrome).[1029]
Smoking (nicotine).[1030]
Social anxiety disorder.[1031]
Soft tissue sarcomas.[1032]
Somatization disorder.[1033]
Sore throat.[1034]
Spasmodic dysphonia (laryngeal dystonia).[1035]
Spasms.[1036]
Spinal cord disease.[1037]
Spinal cord injury.[1038]
Spleen issues.[1039]
Staphylococcus aureus.[1040]
Sternum, pain on touching.[1041]
Stillbirth.[1042]
Still's syndrome (or disease).[1043]
Stomach ache.[1044]
Stomach cancer.[1045]
Stomach ulcer.[1046]
Streptococcus pyogenes.[1047]
Stroke.[1048]
Stuttering.[1049]
Subacromial pain syndrome.[1050]
Subcutaneous cysts.[1051]
Sudden infant death syndrome (SIDS).[1052]
Sudeck's syndrome.[1053]
Suicidal thoughts, tendencies, ideations, or attempts.[1054]
Sunburn, easily.[1055]
Supraventricular tachycardia.[1056]
Susceptibility to contagions.[1057]
Sweaty head area (hyperhidrosis).[1058]
Swine flu (H1N1).[1059]
Swollen glands.[1060]
Syllogomania (hoarding syndrome).[1061]
Syndromic hidradenitis suppurativa.[1062]
Syndromic hydrocephalus.[1063]
Syndrome of inappropriate antidiuretic hormone (SIADH).[1064]
Synovitis.[1065]
Systemic lupus erythematosus (SLE).[1066]
Systemic sclerosis (scleroderma).[1067]

Tachycardia.[1068]
Takayasu's arteritis.[1069]
Takotsubo syndrome.[1070]
Taste impairment.[1071]
TB (tuberculosis).[1072]
Technology addiction.[1073]
Teeth, buck (overbite).[1074]
Teeth, loose.[1075]
Teeth problems (and in children late development of teeth).[1076]
Teeth, weakened teeth that crack, break, or shatter.[1077]
Tendon pain.[1078]
Tennis elbow (lateral epicondylitis).[1079]
Testicular cancer.[1080]
Testosterone issues.[1081]
Tetany syndrome.[1082]
Thalassemia.[1083]
Thrombocytopenia.[1084]
Thrombophilia.[1085]
Thrombosis.[1086]
Thrush.[1087]
Thyroid cancer.[1088]
Thyroid disease.[1089]
TIA (transient ischaemic attack).[1090]
Tibia, pain on touching.[1091]
Timothy syndrome.[1092]
Tinea capitis (ringworm).[1093]
Tinea corporis.[1094]
Tinea incognito.[1095]
Tingling hands or feet ("pins and needles").[1096]
Tinnitus.[1097]
Toenail fungus.[1098]
Tonsillitis.[1099]
Tooth cavities.[1100]
Tooth decay.[1101]
Tooth loss.[1102]
Tourette's syndrome.[1103]
Transgenderism.[1104]
Transexualism.[1105]
Transient ischaemic attack (TIA).[1106]

Transverse myelitis.[1107]
Tremors.[1108]
Trichobezoar syndrome (Rapunzel syndrome).[1109]
Trichomonas infection.[1110]
Trichorhinophalangeal syndrome.[1111]
Trichotillomania.[1112]
Trigeminal neuralgia.[1113]
Trousseau's syndrome.[1114]
Tuberculosis (TB).[1115]
Tuberous sclerosis.[1116]
Tumor-induced osteomalacia.[1117]
Tyrosinemia.[1118]
Ulcerative colitis.[1119]
Ulcers.[1120]
Underactive thyroid.[1121]
Urethra, issues with the.[1122]
Urinary bladder cancer.[1123]
Urinary incontinence.[1124]
Urinary tract infections (UTIs).[1125]
Urination, frequent night.[1126]
Urolithiasis (kidney stones).[1127]
Urticaria.[1128]
Uterine fibroids.[1129]
Uterine cancer.[1130]
Vaginal cancer.[1131]
Vaginal discharge.[1132]
Vaginitis.[1133]
Vaginosis.[1134]
Varicella zoster virus (chickenpox).[1135]
Varicose veins.[1136]
Vascular diseases.[1137]
Vasculitis.[1138]
Vein inflammation (phlebitis).[1139]
Venous leg ulcer.[1140]
Vernal keratoconjunctivitis.[1141]
Vertigo.[1142]
Vibrio cholerae (cholera).[1143]
Violence behaviors.[1144]
Viral infections.[1145]
Viruses.[1146]

Vision, day and night, blurred.[1147]
Vitiligo.[1148]
Voice (vocal) issues.[1149]
Von Hippel-Lindau Disease.[1150]
Von Willebrand disease.[1151]
Vulvar cancer.[1152]
Walking, delayed in children.[1153]
Warts.[1154]
Weakness in shoulders, upper arms, thighs, hips, or legs
    (when in hips or legs can cause waddling).[1155]
Weight gain (excessive).[1156]
Weight loss (excessive).[1157]
Weill-Marchesani syndrome.[1158]
West's syndrome.[1159]
Whipple's disease.[1160]
White spot syndrome.[1161]
Whooping cough.[1162]
Wiedemann-Steiner Syndrome.[1163]
Williams Syndrome.[1164]
Williams-Beuren syndrome.[1165]
Wilms' tumor.[1166]
Wilson disease.[1167]
Winter season.[1168]
Withdrawal, from society.[1169]
Wolff-Parkinson-White syndrome.[1170]
Wolman disease.[1171]
Worry.[1172]
Wound healing, slow.[1173]
Zellweger spectrum disorder.[1174]
Zika virus.[1175]

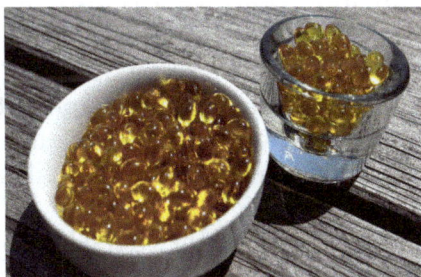

Photograph by Lochlainn Seabrook. Copyright © Lochlainn Seabrook.

YOU ARE PROBABLY A VICTIM OF D DEFICIENCY

Nearly every disease and health concern in the above list has been found to either be caused (in part or fully) by a vitamin D deficiency, to respond favorably to vitamin D therapy, or to be wholly prevented by having the proper amount of vitamin D circulating in the body. (In a few rare cases the illness listed is merely associated with vitamin D in some way, or its connection to vitamin D is assumed but still being studied by medical researchers and laboratories.)

If you have one or more of the conditions listed here, you are quite likely to have a vitamin D deficiency, or an imbalance of some kind related to vitamin D. As I mentioned earlier, vitamin D is so closely linked with every cell, with every physical organ, and nearly every biological process that even if you have a condition that is *not* on this list, it is almost certainly connected to vitamin D in one way or another.

If so, and I cannot stress this enough, it is recommended that you contact your medical care practitioner—preferably one with a background in food science, nutrition, health, fitness, and/or diet.

WHAT TO TRUST & WHAT NOT TO TRUST

Please do not put your full faith in me or the information in this book. *This information is only meant to be a jumping off point for you.* Educate yourself. Do your own research. Follow up on your own hunches and leads. If something resonates with you, pursue it. See where it leads.

A good place to start is the NIH's National Library of Medicine website (better known as "Pub Med"), where as of August 2024 I found over 106,000 articles on or related to vitamin D.[1176] Though quite conventional in its approach to medicine and nutrition, Pub Med is also very thorough in presenting the many varied *mainstream* studies and views related to vitamin D, most which, encouragingly, support the findings of natural and alternative medical practitioners—with only a few exceptions. If you dig deep enough you will find both *complimentary* and even *alternative* medical material related to vitamin D3 on Pub Med.

Read and study, and decide for yourself what is logical and trustworthy and what is not. It is your body and your health.

CHAPTER 4
GETTING HEALTHY

THE GOSPEL OF GOOD HEALTH

Though it is not at all the goal of this book to dictate your personal lifestyle, nor promote a specific diet or nutritional ideology—but merely to educate the public on the importance of vitamin D—as a health researcher and educator it would be irresponsible of me not to take a moment to preach the Gospel of Good Health. For all of the vitamin D therapy in the world will not help you if you are sabotaging your mind and body by sitting inside all day, overeating, abusing drugs, or consuming junk food.

After all, your vitamin D deficiency did not occur by accident, nor did it suddenly appear out of nowhere. It was created through your way of life over a period of many months, or more likely, many years or even decades. Therefore one cannot expect dramatic results from vitamin D therapy without first laying a firm foundation for a future healthy life—complete with the proper levels of circulating vitamin D3 (along with other vital co-factors) in your body.

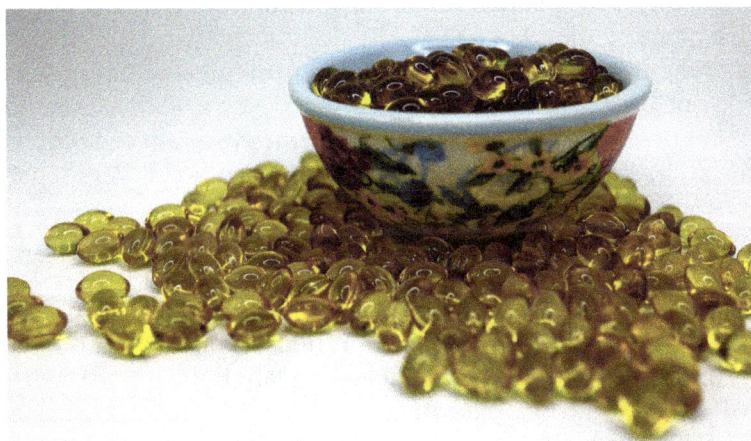

Photograph by Lochlainn Seabrook. Copyright © Lochlainn Seabrook.

CREATING HEALTH VIA A HEALTHY LIFESTYLE

Where to begin? If you want to increase both your health span and your life span, this will not happen by magic. Health, especially as you age, requires attention, effort, discipline, knowledge, and in most cases hard work, if it is to be maintained at maximum levels. Thus, almost without exception, nearly every single health problem discussed in this book (and even most of those that are not), will benefit if you make even one of the following basic changes in your lifestyle:

Lose the extra weight (obesity causes *preventable* diseases).[1177]
Avoid smoking (causes dozens of *preventable* diseases).[1178]
Avoid alcohol (causes dozens of *preventable* diseases).[1179]
Avoid soft drinks (causes dozens of *preventable* diseases).[1180]
Avoid drinking coffee (especially pregnant women).[1181]
Avoid unfiltered tap water.
Use cast-iron and stainless steel cookware (many health authorities advise caution when it comes to both aluminum and all "non-stick" cookware in general).
Avoid foods and drinks stored, sold, or bottled in plastic (microplastics, which seep into foods stored in plastic containers—particularly when heated—are a new and nearly omnipresent health hazard).
Avoid white sugar products. Use natural sweeteners.
Avoid white flour products. Use whole grain products.
Cut down on carbohydrates. (For those with weight- and/or carb-related health concerns, consider the Keto diet or the carnivore diet.)
Fast whenever possible (skip one or more meals a day) to give your body a periodic rest. (Lowering caloric consumption has been shown to lengthen and improve quality of life.)[1182]
Eat fresh, organic, natural meats, dairy products, vegetables, spices, nuts, and seeds whenever possible.
Avoid inorganic foods (those sprayed with or containing chemicals, additives, preservatives, colorings, etc.).
Avoid genetically modified foods, known as GMO, an acronym for "genetically modified organism." (Look for the term non-GMO on packaging labels.)
Not all "health foods" are necessarily healthy: spinach, wheat germ, and almonds, for example, long touted for their

"amazing health benefits," contain a substance called *oxalates*, which can be nothing short of poisonous to certain individuals.[1183]

Another problematic food item is the *lectin*, a type of protein that binds to certain carbohydrates, and which in some people can cause grave digestive disturbances. Foods like peanuts, raw whole grains, tomatoes, potatoes, and raw kidney beans, all contain various levels of lectins that may be hazardous to one's health.[1184]

Another dubious food group is the nightshade family, which includes peppers, white and red potatoes, tobacco, red spices, tomatoes, and eggplant. The nightshades contain alkaloids, which includes a dangerous natural pesticide called *solanine*, that some claim can cause inflammation, digestive problems, arthritic pain, exacerbation of chronic health conditions, and other major medical issues. On the other hand, both nightshades, and even alkaloids themselves, provide a number of health benefits.[1185]

Educate yourself on these important topics.

Avoid snacking between meals.

Avoid overeating. (Leave the table before you are full.)

Avoid processed foods. Make your own meals—from scratch.

Use only sea salt, Celtic or Himalayan sea salt on your food.

Use only olive oil, coconut oil, or avocado oil on your food and for cooking. Avoid vegetable oils, seed oils, and saturated oils, which many health practitioners consider "absolutely poisonous." Natural butter, ghee, and tallow are also excellent health-giving types of oils.

Eat antioxidant-rich foods, such as fresh or frozen blueberries.

Consider taking a daily multivitamin-mineral supplement, since it is essentially impossible to get enough nutrients from food and sunlight (vitamin D). Make sure your supplements are high quality (that is, natural and food-based) and manufactured by a reputable company.

Eat (small) fish species (small to avoid mercury), or fish-oil supplements, and other foods rich in omega-3 fatty acids.

Stay hydrated during the day by consuming pure filtered water.

If you are over 50 do not drink liquids with your meals (wait
  until one hour *after* eating), and cut down, or cut out,
  spicy foods altogether.

If you have symptoms of ailments not discussed in this book,
  you may have food allergies, or perhaps something far
  more serious. Speak to your doctor about your symptoms
  and getting tested. Note that, as mentioned earlier, many
  food allergies can be and are connected to a vitamin D
  deficiency.

Stay active and fit. Get on a doctor-approved daily exercise
  program suited to your age, weight, and lifestyle.
  Incorporate both aerobic and anaerobic exercises. *Vigorous*
  daily exercise has been shown to lengthen and improve life
  quality, and, in some cases, even reverse the aging
  process.[1186]

Meditate, and/or learn how to manage stress.

Pray for spiritual guidance concerning your health issues. A
  little faith in the Unseen goes a long way, as even some
  conventional doctors are now beginning to realize and
  accept.

Develop a wholesome positive attitude toward life. According
  to Jesus, along with many other great spiritual healers and
  leaders throughout history, thoughts become things. Thus,
  as "like attracts like," we must take care to think about only
  those things we want to manifest in our lives (see e.g.,
  Matthew 21:22; Mark 11:24). Healthy thoughts tend to
  lead to healthy outcomes. Toxic thoughts tend to lead to
  further health complications.[1187]

YOUR HEALTH IS *YOUR* RESPONSIBILITY

Many mainstream doctors will scoff at most if not all of my recommendations. I accept such differences in opinion. However, since your health is ultimately *your* responsibility and *not* your doctor's, as always, I encourage you to do your own health research

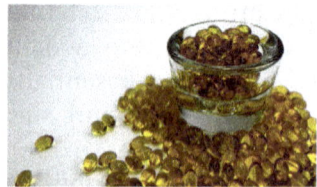

Photograph by Lochlainn Seabrook. Copyright © Lochlainn Seabrook.

and not rely on any one source, including this book. No one
will ever care about your health as much as you do!

Chapter 5
VITAMIN D: IN SUMMARY

A RECAP OF IMPORTANT POINTS
Understandably, for most people, learning about the information in this book will be both wonderful and exciting. Indeed, the "good news" about vitamin D and its relationship to nearly every human ailment is nothing short of miraculous, and most will be impatient to begin on their healing path. For those already in the starting gate, here again is the nonconventional medical or natural health RDA for adults:

DAILY MAINTENANCE DOSE
Vitamin D: 10,000 IU (250 mcg/0.25 mg).
Magnesium: 400 mg.
Vitamin K2: 100 mcg.[1188]

I would caution my readers, however, to go slowly and be patient. Though some people experience rapid transformations after correcting their maintenance vitamin D dose, or getting on a mega-therapeutic vitamin D regimen, some health changes will be more subtle, taking months or even years to physically manifest. Even then there is never a guarantee when it comes to health, as doctors, both conventional and alternative, are always quick to point out.

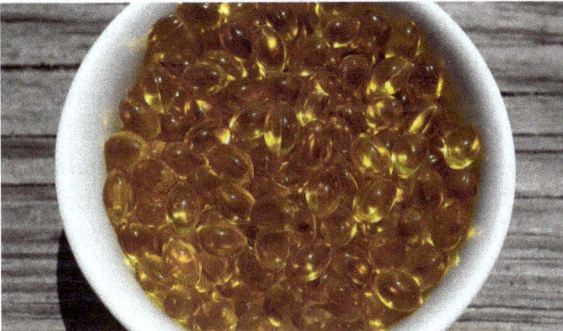

Photograph by Lochlainn Seabrook. Copyright © Lochlainn Seabrook.

Like life itself, health is an endless journey. For everyday our bodies are changing and remodeling at a cellular level due to both the activities of daily life and the aging process. Inevitably this means that our need for vitamin D, as well as our blood serum vitamin D level, will both fluctuate; not only from month to month, but from year to year, as we age and our body, diet, and lifestyle change with time. This emphasizes the importance of staying vigilant when it comes to vitamin D intake, blood testing, and possible signs of a either vitamin D deficiency (hypovitaminosis D) or the much rarer problem of vitamin D toxicity (hypervitaminosis D).

In summation: If you have a single ailment listed in Chapter 3, you are highly likely to have a vitamin D deficiency. A certain percentage of my readers will have a *severe* vitamin D deficiency, with a cascade of obvious health problems and even life-threatening diseases flowing from it. Due to the massive vitamin D deficiency crisis plaguing the world at the moment, even if your health condition is not listed in this book, there is nearly a 100 percent chance that you are deficient in vitamin D, for *most diseases are interconnected in some way—not only to each other, but to vitamin D as well.* Remember: By some estimates, 97 percent of the global population has a vitamin D deficiency.[1189] I was once a part of it. It is likely you are too.

This book, along with your doctor's guidance—whether conventional, alternative, or complimentary—should be able to assist you in determining if and where you fit in on the vitamin D deficiency scale, and what can and needs to be done about it.

As this book is only meant to be a primer on the vast and vital science of vitamin D, after reading it I encourage you to continue your quest for optimal health through your own research and study. It is never too late to get healthy. If you can reach the very attainable goal of getting the proper amount of daily vitamin D, many health professionals believe that it will help you live a longer, happier, better quality life.

Thousands have done just that by learning the secrets of the all-powerful hormone known as vitamin D. You can too!

The End

APPENDICES

*Congressional Statements Concerning
the Proposed 1973 FDA Regulations*

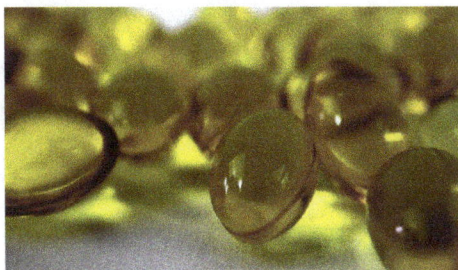

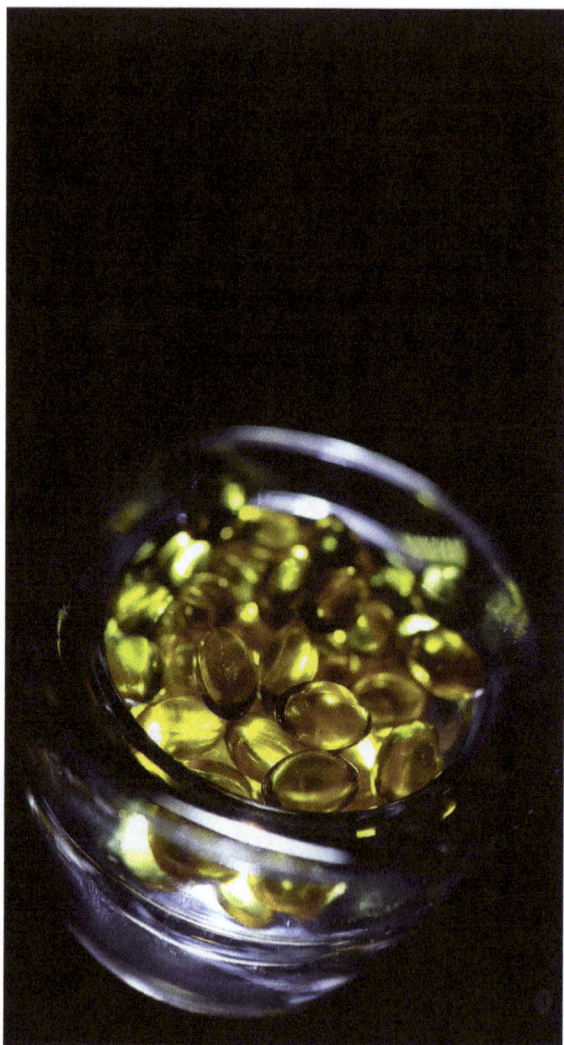

Photograph by Lochlainn Seabrook. Copyright © Lochlainn Seabrook.

APPENDIX A

Address of Democratic Representative William Randall of Missouri before the U.S. House of Representatives regarding the socialistic-style "Food Supplement Amendment of 1973," October 29, 1973.

It is a pleasure to have the opportunity to appear before the Public Health and Environmental Subcommittee of the Interstate and Foreign Commerce Committee today regarding [the bipartisan bill] H.R. 643 (and now H.R. 10093)[1190] referred to as the "Food Supplement Amendment of 1973." I am also appearing on behalf of my own bill, H.R. 11247, which I introduced because quite frankly, some errors were discovered in both [California Republican Representative] Mr. [Craig] Hosmer's initial bill and my own previous bill.[1191]

Of course, like nearly every other member of Congress, I have the privilege of representing approximately one-half million constituents, and I can't recall any matter which has provoked a larger outpouring of mail from my constituents. As we here today know, there has been a sustained public uproar over the Food and Drug Administration's new regulations which set potency limits for vitamins and food supplements.

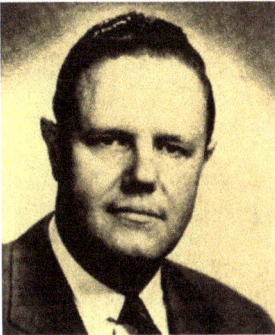

Rep. William Randall.

I know in many of these crusades, a public official receives countless form letters. But this case is different. Speaking from my own personal experience, we have received some form letters but most of the hundreds of letters that have poured into my office over the past year were handwritten and expressed the genuine concern of thousands of ordinary people.

I know I am speaking for myself and I suspect many other members of the House of Representatives when I say we are sympathetic with the desire of the Food and Drug Administration [FDA] to protect consumers from being misled into purchasing dietary supplements which are either valueless or might pose a threat to their health. However, at the heart of this issue is the question of whether vitamins should be regarded as a food substance or a drug; and in this connection, whether the FDA has the authority to control the sale of vitamins and mineral supplements which have not been conclusively proven to be harmful to one's health. In other words, do the new FDA regulations usurp the rights of the consumer?

The FDA regulations are aimed particularly at controlling excessive use of vitamin A and vitamin D, for it has been demonstrated that massive doses of these two substances can be extremely harmful and in some cases deadly. I have no quarrel with the FDA over their right to protect the public from life-threatening substances, however I do disagree with the seemingly arbitrary limits that the FDA has affixed to these two vitamins. For example, although the FDA has set a single limit for both adults and children with respect to vitamins A and D, many medical experts have confirmed that higher levels would be safe and suitable for adults while lower levels should be recommended for children.

To further illustrate the lack of scientific merit of the FDA limits, I would like to note for the benefit of the Committee that two slices of calves liver generally contain three to four times as much vitamin A as the FDA finds permissible, and even a bunch of carrots exceeds the FDA-dictated maximum level. Does this mean that it will require a prescription to buy carrots at the market?

My objections to the new FDA regulations, therefore, is this: why does the Food and Drug Administration persist in maintaining that it is necessary to regulate all vitamins and dietary supplements in order to protect the public from a few? It is my belief that the FDA must differentiate between toxic and non-toxic supplements, and its regulations should cover only the former. In this connection, existing law gives the FDA all the authority it needs to protect the consumer from excessive dosages of substances that might be harmful.

If conclusive evidence can be produced which suggests that certain vitamins in large dosages are so harmful that they should be prescribed by a physician, such control must be accepted. However, if conclusive evidence is not available, the public should be permitted to judge for itself whether or not certain food supplements are necessary and beneficial.

Moreover, I believe that the abuses in the dietary supplement field that originally promoted the imposition of FDA regulations can best and most effectively be corrected by promoting complete disclosatory labeling. The ingredients, nutritive value, recommended dosage, and other dietary information should be plainly printed on the label or package. Once the consumer is fully and accurately informed as to exactly what the product contains he can make a rational decision whether or not to purchase it.

It should also be noted that the all-encompassing FDA regulations will necessitate that many vitamins be sold in smaller amounts in order to comply with arbitrary FDA recommended dosages. This will most assuredly make them more expensive. One estimate has suggested that vitamins may well cost four or five times as much as a consequence, thus denying many consumers—particularly the elderly and those with limited incomes—from adequately fulfilling their nutritional needs and desires.

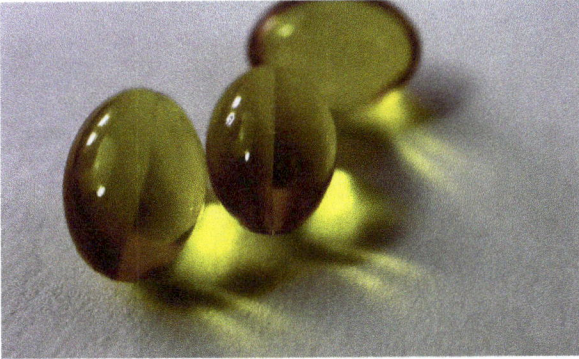

Photograph by Lochlainn Seabrook. Copyright © Lochlainn Seabrook.

In conclusion, this entire controversy over the FDA regulations is a part of a larger problem. Perhaps one of the greatest challenges of our era is to make government work for the people rather than against them. Our society has become so complex and interdependent that the government [has become evermore socialistic, and] has unfortunately intruded into every aspect of our daily existence. To my way of thinking, the role of government is not to deprive people of responsibility, but to encourage them to act responsibly. It is not to dictate to them, but to serve them. The men and women of this nation are not fools who need to be taken by the hand and guided through life by the Federal government. Thus, I believe that so long as the consumer is provided with complete information as to what he or she is purchasing, the consumer is both competent and entitled to determine his or her own best nutritional needs.

I reject the assumption contained in the FDA regulations that the Food and Drug Administration has a right and responsibility to prevent consumers—who are in full possession of disclosatory information—from making a choice regarding non-toxic dietary supplements which the Agency thinks is "irrational" or "unwise." As I have noted on many occasions, we have strict regulations that require that poisons be clearly labeled; but as far as I know there has never been a statute passed that prohibits anyone from taking poison. In other words, when the labeling is on the bottle, the responsibility shifts to the other side, to the consumer.

For the past ten years, we have been successful in frustrating the FDA's campaign to limit the potency and formulation of dietary supplements. However, because of the FDA's recent action giving final approval to restrictive new regulations, the time has come for Congress to take firm action to insure the rights and freedom of the consumer. In closing, let me express, on behalf of my many constituents who wrote me regarding this controversial issue, our appreciation for the Committee's willingness to hold these hearings.[1192]

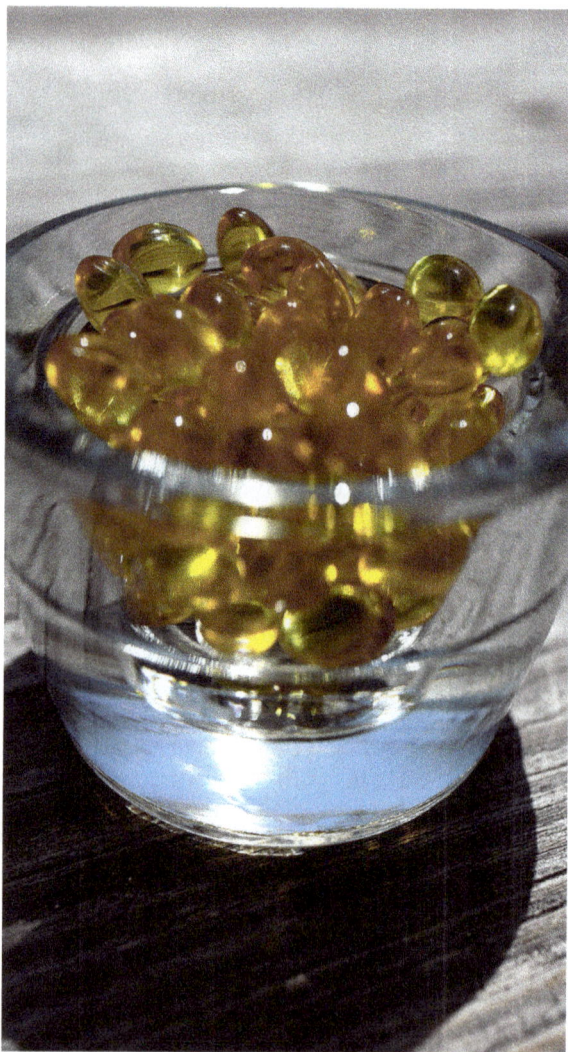

Photograph by Lochlainn Seabrook. Copyright © Lochlainn Seabrook.

APPENDIX B

Statement of Hon. Frank Annunzio, a Democratic representative in Congress from the state of Illinois, 1973.

Mr. Chairman, on August 2, after more than a decade of dispute, the Food and Drug Administration issued regulations restricting the marketing of vitamin and mineral products. Since the FDA first proposed these regulations in January of this year, congressional offices have been inundated by mail protesting such action. The sources of the complaints have been varied; seldom does regulatory action generate such heavy criticism from both the consumer and industry.

Both interests have every right to complain. At a time when numerous studies are showing gross deficiencies in the vitamin and mineral intake of Americans, the FDA has taken action to decrease the availability of food supplements. Under the new regulation, certain supplements are now classified as drugs rather than foods. The costly marketing requirements for drugs will drive up prices, making the vitamin-mineral products least available to those who need them most.

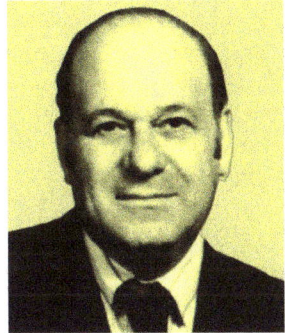

Rep. Frank Annunzio.

Those supplements which are now arbitrarily classified as drugs either have dosage levels higher on a per unit basis than those prescribed by the FDA regulation, or they have combinations of supplements other than those allowed. In the case of two vitamins, A and D, dosage levels over a certain amount will now be available only by prescription. Eventually, even more of the supplements may be placed on prescription-only status. An advisory review panel has been requested to provide its advice on the dividing line between over-the-counter and prescription drugs.

I can see no reason for the FDA to promulgate such regulations. Most vitamins and minerals present no danger to the consumer, indeed, they may be highly beneficial. If some of the vitamins are hazardous at high levels, as may be the case for the vitamins A and D, they should be limited. However, criticism has poured from academic, consumer, and industry sources, protesting the levels prescribed are far too low—400 IU for vitamin D and 10,000 IU for vitamin A.

Considering the present level of knowledge regarding the need for vitamin and mineral supplements, whether or not a benefit can be derived from high potency supplements seems to be a very subjective decision. But regardless of the availability or lack of benefits, the consumer has every right to purchase food supplements at dosage levels he desires as long as they are unadulterated, correctly labeled, and present no hazard to health. The FDA seems to have made a value judgment that consumers are wasting their money on useless supplements. It is not within the legislative mandate of the FDA to regulate how the consumer spends his money; only to protect his safety.

In an attempt to stop this abuse of authority, I have sponsored legislation which would require the FDA to prove any vitamin or mineral (synthetic or natural) is "intrinsically injurious to health in the recommended dosage," before restricting its dosage level of [or?] requiring a warning label. H.R. 643 would prohibit the FDA from arbitrarily controlling what goes into vitamin-mineral supplements. In those instances where a high potency supplement does pose a threat to health, the FDA would be free to impose limits on the dosage strengths or require a warning label.

Mr. Chairman, I have sponsored this amendment to the Federal Food, Drug and Cosmetic Act in the firm belief that its passage is imperative if we are to protect the rights not only of the manufacturers, but of the consumer. I am, therefore, delighted that these hearings are being held and urge that early and favorable action be taken by the committee and the Congress.[1193]

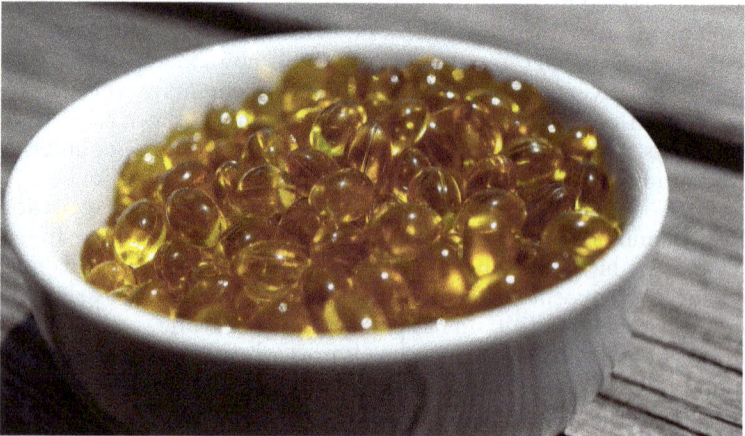

Photograph by Lochlainn Seabrook. Copyright © Lochlainn Seabrook.

APPENDIX C

Statement of Hon. Clarence E. Miller, a Republican representative
in Congress from the state of Ohio, 1973.

Mr. Chairman, I appreciate having this opportunity to express my
support for H.R. 643 and commend the committee for holding these
hearings on a matter in which there is such an overwhelming public and
congressional interest.

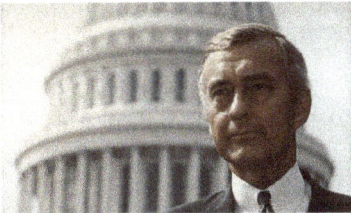

Rep. Clarence E. Miller.

The Food and Drug
Administration ended a decade of
controversy on January 19 this year
when it issued final orders restricting
the sale of vitamins and dietary
supplements. Beginning next year,
19 vitamins and minerals at levels in
excess of 150 percent of the
recommended daily allowance will
be classified as drugs, labeled as such,
and sold only by prescription. Any
enriched or fortified food must be elaborately labeled to specify exact
RDA percentages of vitamins and minerals.

Admittedly, I am no nutritionist—in fact, I am probably one of the
lay people the FDA says is incapable of determining whether they have
vitamin or mineral deficiencies—but a reading of the FDA regulations
and their justifications led me to believe that neither is the FDA. While
the FDA's motives may be noble and well intentioned, as most
bureaucracies are these days, the uneasy fact is that the scientific base for
its conclusion is shaky and the broad sweep of its proposals has far
exceeded its statutory authority to protect the public from fraud and
contamination.

My staff and I have waded through the lengthy FDA proposal as well
as other scientific documents relating to nutrition. I am frank to admit
we have come across no preponderance of scientific evidence to prove
[the] FDA's claim that vitamins and food supplements are hazardous to
health in any quantity.

The Food and Drug Administration has made some very broad
assumptions to support their case:

> "Loss of nutrients from the ordinary effects of cooking,
> processing, transportation, and storage has not
> significantly impaired the nutritional quality" . . . "Many
> dietary supplements are nutritionally irrational" . . .

"Vitamin or mineral deficiencies are unrelated to . . . tiredness, nervousness, and rundown condition" . . . "It is inaccurate to state that the quality of soil in the United States causes abnormally low concentrations of vitamins and minerals in the food supply produced in this country."

These statements are not established facts in the scientific community. They are propositions and opinion that must await a definitive verdict, but in a few short weeks regulations will give them the full force of law.

According to the FDA, the regulations will reduce "consumer confusion." [The] FDA apparently has assumed unto itself the role of national shopper and will impose its own market judgment on all the people. Obviously, this goes beyond its function of promoting safety.

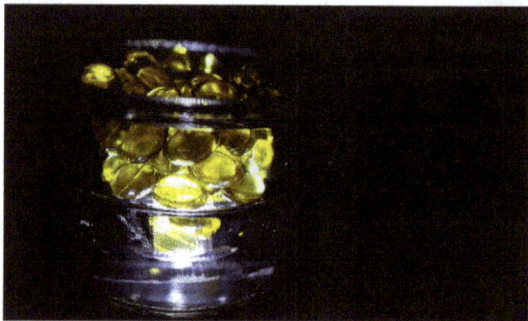

Photograph by Lochlainn Seabrook. Copyright © Lochlainn Seabrook.

But, more importantly to me, it is the kind of arrogance that is particularly objectionable in a Washington bureaucracy.

[The] FDA has no monopoly on the truth, nor is it omniscient. It has no inherent right to interfere with the freedom of choice among millions of Americans who deem it necessary to supplement a diet they deem inadequate. Surely FDA has better, more proper things to do on behalf of the American people than merely making it less convenient and more expensive to buy vitamins and minerals.

H.R. 643, the so-called Hosmer bill of which I am a cosponsor, is a reasonable proposal to reassert the legislative function of the Congress in an area we seem to have long ago abandoned. H.R. 643 will bar the FDA from denying people the right to buy vitamins and other safe food without impairing its statutory authority to protect the public from inherently unsafe or injurious substances.

Obviously, the subcommittee has recognized the wide support for this legislation, and I hope it will act expeditiously and favorably in reporting to the full committee.[1194]

APPENDIX D

Statement of Hon. Leo J. Ryan, a Democratic representative in Congress from the state of California, 1973.

Mr. Chairman, time and time again, the Congress is called upon to right a wrong perpetrated on an unsuspecting public by an overzealous or ill-informed agency of the Federal Government. I testify today in support of legislation that would correct a particularly meddlesome ruling about to be thrust on the public by the Food and Drug Administration. The promulgation of these new regulations represents an 11-year effort by the FDA to make harmless vitamin and mineral products less freely available to consumers. Guidelines to restrict the contents and dosages of food supplements have been proposed several times since 1962, each time meeting massive criticism from consumers. This instance is no different, except that the regulations are now final and will become effective January 24.

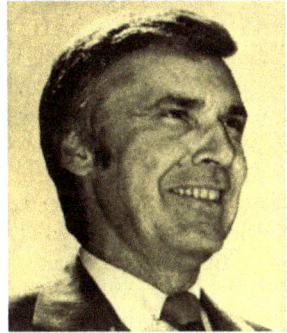

Rep. Leo J. Ryan.

These regulations have generated an unbelievable volume of letters from concerned citizens who fear that they will no longer be able to obtain many of their favorite food supplements without a prescription, or anticipate that the new regulations will increase the cost of all vitamin mineral products. It is my judgment that their fears are entirely justified.

These new regulations would allow food supplements to contain only a very small number of vitamins and minerals. In addition, the dosage levels of these nutrients are not allowed to exceed extremely low levels. All other combinations and dosage levels of vitamin and mineral products, with two exceptions, would be available only as over-the-counter drugs. These two exceptions are vitamins A and D. The new regulations require that all products which contain these two vitamins, in dosage units over certain levels, to be sold only as prescription drugs.

These low levels have been heavily criticized by numerous authorities in the field of nutrition. For example, Dr. Linus Pauling, winner of the 1962 Nobel Prize for Chemistry, has concluded that the optimum daily intake of vitamin A is 21½ times that allowed by the Food and Drug Administration. Further, Dr. Pauling believes that there is very little danger of hypervitaminosis [overdosing] with vitamin A. The maximum dosage allowed by the FDA for the vitamin D is also considered too low. Ultimately, as consumers fear, many other supplements may be available only by prescription.

Experience demonstrates that many of these vitamins and minerals will no longer be

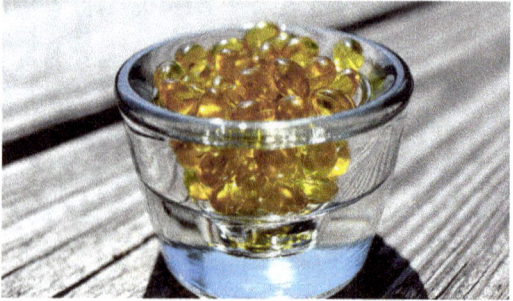

Photograph by Lochlainn Seabrook. Copyright © Lochlainn Seabrook.

known by their generic term. They will take on whatever trade name that the manufacturer's best marketing people can concoct to insure that their vitamins are prescribed by the physicians around the country. Thus, the physicians when writing their prescriptions will be able to choose between Delight Dollops of D Vitamin or Super-D-Doodle-D-Vitamin.

As we have seen in the past, many drugs that lose their generic names in favor of a trade name increase in cost astronomically. It is not difficult to imagine what will happen to the cost of food supplements and vitamins when they are designated as prescription drugs. The consumer will have to pay for the costly labeling and marketing requirements for prescription drugs, plus the doctor's fee to get the prescription.

I would like to point out at this time that I do not wish to be critical of the fine work the FDA has done in protecting the country from dangerous and unsafe drugs. I do, however, challenge the FDA to demonstrate the harm or even the decreased efficacy caused by vitamins or other food supplements, even close to the levels that the Food and Drug Administration wishes to regulate them as though they were "dangerous drugs."

In an effort to stop such arbitrary action on the part of the FDA, I would urge the committee to take speedy action on H.R. 643. This type of legislation has been introduced in the past three Congresses, to limit the authority of the Food and Drug Administration. If action is not taken this year, the regulations will be final and will become effective January 1974. This legislation would require the FDA to show that any synthetic or natural vitamin mineral, or other food supplement, is "intrinsically injurious to health" before limiting its use. I do not think it is unreasonable that this requirement be placed on the FDA. Moreover, I think it is an absolute necessity in order to protect the American consumer from an unrealistic and totally unreasonable burden in their pursuit of a healthy state of being.[1195]

APPENDIX E

Statement of Hon. James Abdnor, a Republican representative in Congress from the state of South Dakota, 1973.

Mr. Chairman, members of the Subcommittee on Public Health and the Environment, thank you for giving me the opportunity to submit testimony in opposition to the Food and Drug Administration's regulations for dietary food supplements. My statement is in support of H.R. 643 providing for corrective measures on proposals greatly and questionably restricting the potency of over-the-counter vitamin and mineral supplements.

I am not an expert on health requirements, nor am I a campaigning nutritionist. I cannot make claims of absolute knowledge about vitamin and mineral needs, nor can I disclaim with authority the findings of the FDA's "extensive" research into potency requirements, and thusly, allowances. I can only point out some highly questionable inconsistencies in the scientific supportive data for the regulations, let alone the questionable intent of the Government to further erode personal freedoms under the guise of "informational" consumer protection.

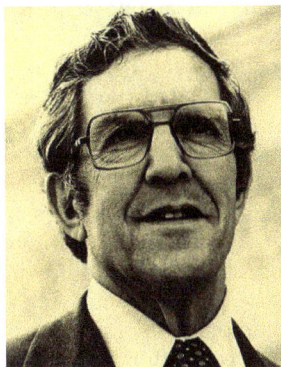

I would first like to commend the FDA on their efforts and desires to improve the nutritional well-being of Americans. This is a fine goal and an objective worth lending our total support and energy, especially when one considers the highly developed food processing technology of our Nation. I have no arguments with the regulations dealing with food labeling and applaud the FDA for coming forth with a well designed plan of credibility and implementation. It is our responsibility to see to it that more and better information about a food's nutritional quality gets to the public and that the information is meaningful and usable. It is here that I doubt the reliability of the regulations: meaningful and usable information.

The FDA claims "meaningful and usable" nutritional information is dependent upon the replacement of an outmoded system of measuring nutritional intake and have moved from the "minimum" need to the "recommended" need. This philosophy of "recommended" need is highly visible in the regulations for the allowable levels of potency for dietary supplements, or, have you, vitamins. We would not only no longer have

Rep. James Abdnor.

the terminology of Minimum Daily Requirements, which is proposed to be supplanted by the new terminology of Recommended Daily Allowances, but the allowable potency levels themselves are highly questionable and lack sufficient justification for acceptance and codification as recommendations.

Although some aspects of the dietary supplement regulations are highly meritorious in that "meaningful and usable" information can standardize vitamin-mineral preparation and point out that health is not gained by vitamins alone, others are questionable and leave in doubt the FDA's credibility to carry out their own goals. The regulations allowable potency levels for vitamins A, D, and C recommended by the FDA leaves me to conclude that informational nutrition objectives gave way to administrative arbitrariness with little justification in known levels of vitamin toxicity.

I do not want to dwell here upon the many inconsistent findings of research into the toxic levels of vitamins A and D, nor is it necessary to argue myths and nutritional psychosis. I would simply like to ask why the FDA set the potency level for vitamin A at one-tenth of the lowest level known toxicity level. I would also like to ask why the FDA set the potency level for vitamin D at one-fifth the lowest known toxicity level. These levels appear to be nothing but arbitrary figures, and I object to such neglect of reasonable responsibility in carrying out the intent of the Federal Food, Drug, and Cosmetic Act.

Photograph by Lochlainn Seabrook. Copyright © Lochlainn Seabrook.

I have a great deal of respect for the intent and purpose of FDA, but administrative overzealousness is apparent in their regulations of dietary supplements. It is our responsibility as legislators to restrain that zealousness and provide guidelines whereby we avoid the pending encroachments of certain rights and freedoms while yet maintaining all intents and purposes of nutritional information and protection.

I have seen the unreasonable infringement of rights and freedoms in laws passed out of passion and high emotions before. Regardless of our moral quest in safeguarding the public, unreasonable restrictions gradually erode the foundations on which this country was founded.

I urge the subcommittee to act swiftly before the full Interstate and Foreign Commerce Committee in reporting H.R. 643 to the House floor. I can see no harm in restricting vitamin and mineral supplements only to those levels known to be just under the lowest known toxicity level.[1196]

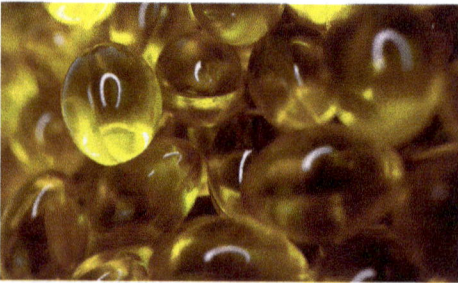

APPENDIX F

Statement of Hon. George M. O'Brien, a Republican representative in Congress from the state of Illinois, 1973.

Mr. Chairman, I appreciate this opportunity to present to the subcommittee my views on the recently issued regulations of the U.S. Food and Drug Administration affecting food supplements. I strongly object to these regulations and respectfully urge this subcommittee to report favorably my bill, H.R. 6170, which would prevent the FDA from interfering in the sale of truthfully labeled vitamin and mineral food supplements for reasons other than safety or fraud.

Because the FDA's deadline for the implementation of these regulations is set for the end of this year this legislation assumes a new urgency and I am most grateful to the subcommittee for scheduling hearings on this matter.

My bill, H.R. 6107, introduced on March 26, is identical to H.R. 643, introduced by Congressman Hosmer of California. It defines food supplements and special dietary uses of food. It also prohibits

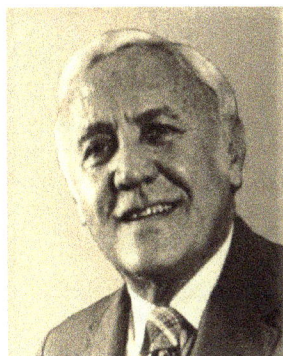

Rep. George M. O'Brien.

FDA limitations on the potency, number, combination, amount, variety, or use of food supplements unless intrinsically injurious to health in the recommended dosage and limits the FDA's authority to require warning labels on food supplements to instances where the recommended dosage is intrinsically injurious to health.

My remarks will be brief. I do not pretend to be an expert on the subject of nutrition. Nor do I wish to act as final arbiter in the lengthy and interminable disputes between the proponents and opponents of natural foods and food supplements.

I do regard myself as something of an expert on the views and needs of the people of the 17th Illinois Congressional District. I have heard from a great many of them on the subject of food supplements and their opinion has been unanimous. The new FDA regulations are bad news.

One does not need to be an expert on nutrition to understand why. The people of my home district believe in freedom of choice. They have confidence in their own and in their fellow man's ability to weigh evidence and to come to a rational conclusion. They resent this effort on the part of the U.S. Food and Drug Administration to make "fact" of opinion and to impede free choice. They are repelled by the idea that a Washington bureaucrat can decree as "fact" that the vitamin content of a food is not significantly affected by its storage, transportation, processing or cooking or by the soil in which it is grown. They are disturbed by the fact that the FDA can give its opinion the force of law and compel adherence to these "facts" under pain of criminal sanction. In their opinion the FDA's new regulations amount to a censorship of ideas and to an unnecessary restriction on the individual's right to eat as he chooses even at the risk of making a mistake.

Research in nutrition is only beginning. Conclusions as to the validity of various nutritional propositions are at best educated guesses. Two hundred years ago bleeding by leeches represented the last word in medical treatment. One can only wonder what the state of medicine would be today if opinions to the contrary had been banned as "mislabeling."

No one questions the right and obligation of the Food and Drug Administration to protect the public from mislabeled goods or from food supplements proven hazardous to one's health. But the FDA's new regulations go far beyond these legitimate ends. They run counter to the concepts of freedom of choice and of free interchange of ideas which are essential to a democratic society.[1197]

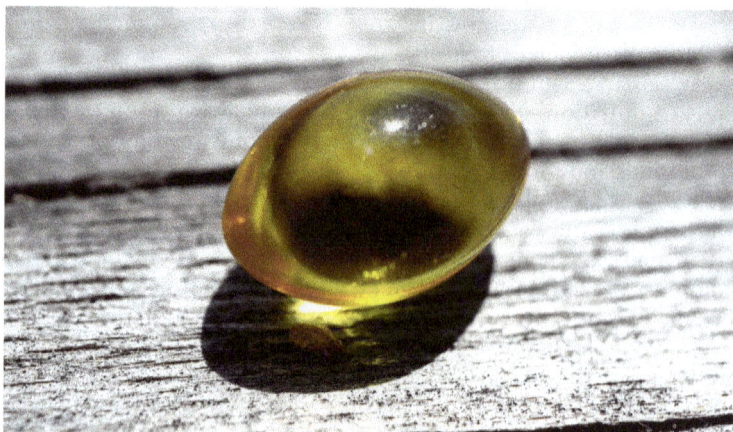

Photograph by Lochlainn Seabrook. Copyright © Lochlainn Seabrook.

NOTES

1. See e.g., Weiss, pp. 360-361.
2. See article: https://pubmed.ncbi.nlm.nih.gov/35934687/.
3. Our bodies cannot make, or even store, some vitamins—such as vitamin C (L-ascorbic acid).
4. Congressional Hearing, p. 872.
5. Mish, s.v. "Vitamin D."
6. See e.g., Somerville, p. 29.
7. Zaidi, p. 18.
8. Ryan, pp. 33-34. Despite the FDA's scientifically untenable stance that "that there is no difference between natural and synthetic vitamins" (Congressional Hearing, p. 877), synthetic vitamins have been known to create serious health problems since at least the 1970s, if not before. See, e.g., Congressional Hearing, pp. 872-874.
9. *Food and Nutrition*, p. 30.
10. *Your Body Can Heal Itself*, p. 352.
11. Congressional Hearing, p. 699.
12. Hausman and Hurley, pp. 99, 270.
13. *Your Body Can Heal Itself*, pp. 41, 316-317, 353.
14. Congressional Hearing, p. 722.
15. Congressional Hearing, p. 636.
16. Zaidi, p. 241.
17. Kaplan and Beech, p. 199.
18. *Encyclopedia Britannica*, s.v. "Vitamin D." Article: https://www.britannica.com/science/vitamin-D. Accessed 4 July 2024. See also article: https://pubchem.ncbi.nlm.nih.gov/compound/1_25-Dihydroxyvitamin-D3.
19. Article: https://www.ncbi.nlm.nih.gov/pmc/articles/PMC6342654/. See also video: "Your Body is Begging for Vitamin D!" YouTube channel: Dr. Eric Berg DC.
20. *Encyclopedia Britannica*, s.v. "Vitamin D." Article: https://www.britannica.com/science/vitamin-D. Accessed 4 July 2024. See also article: https://pubchem.ncbi.nlm.nih.gov/compound/1_25-Dihydroxyvitamin-D3.
21. Webpage: https://pubmed.ncbi.nlm.nih.gov/37371637/.
22. Webpage: https://pubmed.ncbi.nlm.nih.gov/37371637/.
23. Video: "I Might Get Banned for This . . ." YouTube channel: Dr. Eric Berg DC.
24. See video: "Your Body is Begging for Vitamin D!" YouTube channel: Dr. Eric Berg DC.
25. Article: "Vitamin D Receptor Polymorphisms and Cancer." Webpage: https://pubmed.ncbi.nlm.nih.gov/32918214/.
26. Hausman and Hurley, p. 436.
27. Zaidi, p. 10.
28. Bowles, p. 4.
29. Khalsa, p. 160.
30. See *Recommended Dietary Allowances*, passim.
31. Congressional Hearing, pp. 629, 630.
32. Congressional Hearing, p. 630. See also Congressional Hearings, p. 933. In one truly stunning case the FDA claimed that "vitamins and food supplements are hazardous to health in any quantity." Congressional Hearing, p. 773.
33. Congressional Hearing, p. 848.
34. Vitamin D Fact Sheet, NIH government article: https://ods.od.nih.gov/factsheets/VitaminD-HealthProfessional.
35. Congressional Hearing, p. 707.
36. Congressional Hearing, pp. 735-736. For more on these topics see the Appendices.
37. Bowles, pp. 14-15.
38. Khalsa, p. 40.

39. *Bottom Line's 2021 Health Breakthroughs*, p. 247.

40. Khalsa, pp. xii, 40-41.

41. "Writing in 1966, Wallace Marshall, M.D., said that the FDA proposal [of 400 IU daily] was 'based on archaic and highly questionable findings,' and that his work indicated that an intake of 3,000 to 5,000 units of vitamin D a day was perfectly safe." Congressional Hearing, p. 876.

42. See video: "Is it Safe to Take 10,000 IU of Vitamin D3?" YouTube channel: Dr. Eric Berg DC. Also see video: "The Best Way to Optimize Your Absorption of Vitamin D." YouTube channel: The Dr. [Steven] Gundry Podcast.

43. Dowd and Stafford, p. 57.

44. Zaidi, p. 212.

45. Khalsa, pp. 163-164. According to Dr. Alan D. Whanger of Duke University Medical Center: "Some toxic symptoms may appear if 50,000 units of vitamin D is taken daily for several weeks, but usually 10 times that amount is required." That is, 500,000 IU daily. Congressional Hearing, p. 913.

46. See Bowles, passim.

47. Website: https://www.coimbraprotocol.com/the-protocol-1. See also article: https://www.ncbi.nlm.nih.gov/pmc/articles/PMC8058406/.

48. Article: https://pubmed.ncbi.nlm.nih.gov/24246341/.

49. Article: https://pubmed.ncbi.nlm.nih.gov/24246341/.

50. Congressional Hearing, p. 962.

51. Bowles, pp. 156-157. See article: https://pubmed.ncbi.nlm.nih.gov/12514284/. "The Committee of the American Academy of Pediatrics has set the toxic dose of vitamin D at from 1,000 to 3,000 IU *per kilogram of body weight*. Translated into everyday language, that means that 68,000 IU to 2 million IU, for a man of 150 lbs." Congressional Hearing, p. 876.

52. For more on the dangers of synthetic vitamins, see Congressional Hearing, pp. 871-874.

53. Congressional Hearing, p. 876.

54. Zaidi, p. 177.

55. The "stable dose" of 10,000 IU per day is an RDA put forth by former neurologist and now sleep specialist Dr. Stasha Gominak. See Somerville, p. 69.

56. Somerville, pp. 69-71.

57. Khalsa, p. 161; Holick, p. 217.

58. Somerville, p. 69.

59. See e.g., Somerville, pp. 29-30; Holick, pp. 159-160; Khalsa, pp. 156-158.

60. Congressional Hearing, pp. 874, 912.

61. Khalsa, p. 21.

62. Bowles, p. 159.

63. For more on the orthodox medical establishment from several former insiders, see video: "Calley & Casey Means: How Big Pharma Keeps You Sick, and the Dark Truth About Ozempic and the Pill." YouTube channel: Tucker Carlson.

64. For more on this topic see the Appendices.

65. Congressional Hearing, pp. 627, 756. See also my Appendix B.

66. Congressional Hearing, pp. 879-881.

67. See e.g., Congressional Hearing, p. 872.

68. See Bowles, p. 26.

69. Robert F. Kennedy Jr. (born 1954) notes that: "Right now 75 percent of [the] FDA's budget is coming from pharmaceutical companies. That is a perverse incentive." Fox News, August 25, 2024.

70. See *Food and Nutrition*, p. 219.

71. Vitamin D Fact Sheet, NIH government article: https://ods.od.nih.gov/factsheets/VitaminD-HealthProfessional.

72. Holick, p. xxi.

73. Articles: https://www.ncbi.nlm.nih.gov/books/NBK56061/. https://nutritionsource.hsph.harvard.edu/vitamin-d/.

74. Vitamin D Fact Sheet, NIH government article: https://ods.od.nih.gov/factsheets/VitaminD-HealthProfessional.

75. Khalsa, pp. 36-37, 152-153.

76. Congressional Hearing, p. 699.

77. *Bottom Line's 2021 Health Breakthroughs*, pp. 110-111.

78. Website: https://www.nih.gov/about-nih.
79. Vitamin D Fact Sheet, NIH government article: https://ods.od.nih.gov/factsheets/VitaminD-HealthProfessional.
80. Zaidi, p. 20.
81. *Smart Nutrition*, p. 42.
82. Vitamin D Fact Sheet, NIH government article: https://ods.od.nih.gov/factsheets/VitaminD-HealthProfessional.
83. See e.g., Somerville, pp. 60-61.
84. Ryan, p. 22.
85. Bowles, pp. 10, 12.
86. For more on the importance of sunlight to human health, see article: https://articles.mercola.com/sites/articles/archive/2024/08/15/ultraviolet-blood-irradiation.aspx?ui=b7ba10cc52fb2002ce406db13f0ed710b654e3b73c09e60c422ccd7b24eae4f6&sd=20240724&cid_source=dnl&cid_medium=email&cid_content=art1ReadMore&cid=20240815&foDate=false&mid=DM1616155&rid=97484499.
87. Congressional Hearing, p. 962.
88. *Smart Nutrition*, p. 40.
89. *Food and Nutrition*, pp. 30, 150.
90. See video: "The Best Way to Optimize Your Absorption of Vitamin D." YouTube channel: The Dr. [Steven] Gundry Podcast.
91. While researching for this book I came across a new sunscreen technology, a product called "Solar D," which is designed to block harmful sunlight while allowing the synthesis of vitamin D. Visit the company's Website for more information: www.solar-d.com
92. Khalsa, p. 43.
93. For more on the dangers of synthetic vitamins, see Congressional Hearing, pp. 871-874.
94. Zaidi, p. 11.
95. See article: https://www.ncbi.nlm.nih.gov/pmc/articles/PMC6429189/#:~:text=Menaquinone%2D7%20(MK7)%20is%20the%20menaquinone%20of%20fermentative%20origin,K2%20present%20in%20the%20diet.
96. See video: "The Big Lie About Vitamin D." YouTube channel: Dr. Eric Berg.
97. See video: "Is it Safe to Take 10,000 IU of Vitamin D3?" YouTube channel: Dr. Eric Berg DC.
98. See video: "The Unique Benefits of Using Vitamin D and K2 Combined." YouTube channel: Dr. Eric Berg DC.
99. For the magnesium RDAs for children, pregnant women, and breastfeeding women, see article: https://ods.od.nih.gov/factsheets/Magnesium-Consumer/.
100. A 1960s government-sponsored survey "found that only fewer than 200 physicians in the whole country had had nutrition education beyond one semester hour of 'hospital dietetics.'" Congressional Hearing, p. 816.
101. In point of fact: "The whole concept of daily allowances set at a specific figure is . . . open to question, since nutrition has not been incorporated into medical science, vast uncertainty exists with respect to what the human needs may be for any individual nutrients, such as, minerals, amino acids and vitamins." Congressional Hearing, p. 779.
102. See video: "The Best Way to Optimize Your Absorption of Vitamin D." YouTube channel: The Dr. [Steven] Gundry Podcast.
103. *Food and Nutrition*, pp. 30, 59. A new form of vitamin D, dihydroxyvitamin D, has been created for use in treating cancer and other diseases. Unlike ordinary vitamin D, because it does not mobilize calcium, dihydroxyvitamin D will not cause hypercalcemia, and is therefore safe to use in high doses. See *Food and Nutrition*, p. 5.
104. See video: "The Big Lie About Vitamin D." YouTube channel: Dr. Eric Berg.
105. *Smart Nutrition*, p. 42; Congressional Hearing, p. 633.
106. Zaidi, pp. 204-205. See also: https://www.aafp.org/pubs/afp/collections/choosing-wisely/140.html.
107. Ryan, p. 31.
108. For more on animals and vitamin D, see Bowles, p. 14; Ryan, pp. 26-27. For more on natural pet health see Youtube channel: "Dr. Karen Becker." https://www.youtube.com/c/MercolaHealthyPets.
109. Webpage: https://pubmed.ncbi.nlm.nih.gov/38698906/.

110. See article: "The Vitamin D Deficiency Pandemic: Approaches for Diagnosis, Treatment and Prevention," by Michael F. Holick. Webpage: https://pubmed.ncbi.nlm.nih.gov/28516265/.

111. Video: "#1 Vitamin D Danger You Absolutely Must Know!" YouTube channel: Dr. Sten Ekberg.

112. Vitamin D Fact Sheet, NIH government article: https://ods.od.nih.gov/factsheets/VitaminD-HealthProfessional.

113. Somerville, p. 69.

114. Zaidi, p. 20.

115. Guinness, p. 128.

116. *Food and Nutrition*, pp. 30, 79, 358.

117. Bowles, p. 110; see also Zaidi, pp. 15-16.

118. *Smart Nutrition*, p. 41.

119. Video: "#1 Vitamin D Danger You Absolutely Must Know!" YouTube channel: Dr. Sten Ekberg.

120. Article: https://www.universityofcalifornia.edu/news/higher-levels-vitamin-d-correspond-lower-cancer-risk.

121. Khalsa, pp. xi, 81.

122. A UK cancer research center estimates that there are "more than 200 types" of cancer. See https://www.cancerresearchuk.org/about-cancer/what-is-cancer/how-cancer-starts/types-of-cancer#:~:text=For%20example%2C%20nerves%20and%20muscles,of%20cell%20they%20start%20in.

123. See article: https://www.ncbi.nlm.nih.gov/pmc/articles/PMC5764584/#:~:text=The%20anatomical%20disease%20section%20includes,%2C%20muscle%2C%20and%20reproductive%20diseases.

124. An example of bodily remodeling was put forth many years ago by Professor Roger J. Williams, a biochemist at the University of Texas: "Superficially our bones are largely mineral matter—mostly calcium phosphates—and one might suppose that once the skeleton is formed, nutrition of the bone would stop. This is far from true. By the use of 'isotopic tracers' biochemists have found that even in an adult body, the bones are alive; the situation is dynamic rather than static. Bones contain living bone cells which require not only minerals for building bone but all of the other food elements that other living cells need in order to maintain themselves." Congressional Hearing, p. 875.

125. See Congressional Hearings, pp. 874-875.

126. Articles: https://pubmed.ncbi.nlm.nih.gov/26603433/. https://pubmed.ncbi.nlm.nih.gov/34518086/. https://pubmed.ncbi.nlm.nih.gov/34518086/. https://pubmed.ncbi.nlm.nih.gov/27283745/.

127. Articles: https://pubmed.ncbi.nlm.nih.gov/26603433/. https://pubmed.ncbi.nlm.nih.gov/34518086/. https://pubmed.ncbi.nlm.nih.gov/34518086/. https://pubmed.ncbi.nlm.nih.gov/27283745/.

128. Articles: https://pubmed.ncbi.nlm.nih.gov/34766885/. https://pubmed.ncbi.nlm.nih.gov/31757059/. Related article: https://pubmed.ncbi.nlm.nih.gov/31757059/.

129. Articles: https://pubmed.ncbi.nlm.nih.gov/30358967/. https://pubmed.ncbi.nlm.nih.gov/11308051/. https://pubmed.ncbi.nlm.nih.gov/855647/. https://pubmed.ncbi.nlm.nih.gov/15960365/.

130. Articles: https://www.ncbi.nlm.nih.gov/pmc/articles/PMC8215305/. https://www.ncbi.nlm.nih.gov/pmc/articles/PMC9032397/.

131. Article: https://pubmed.ncbi.nlm.nih.gov/29460332/.

132. Article: https://pubmed.ncbi.nlm.nih.gov/30574856/. https://pubmed.ncbi.nlm.nih.gov/36387030/.

133. Articles: https://pubmed.ncbi.nlm.nih.gov/?term=vitamin+d+Acromegaly. https://pubmed.ncbi.nlm.nih.gov/35138562/. https://pubmed.ncbi.nlm.nih.gov/24002366/. https://pubmed.ncbi.nlm.nih.gov/26547217/. https://pubmed.ncbi.nlm.nih.gov/28372721/. https://pubmed.ncbi.nlm.nih.gov/25839036/. https://pubmed.ncbi.nlm.nih.gov/31616375/. https://pubmed.ncbi.nlm.nih.gov/7211102/.

134. Article: https://pubmed.ncbi.nlm.nih.gov/25207381/.

135. Articles: https://pubmed.ncbi.nlm.nih.gov/35160157/. https://pubmed.ncbi.nlm.nih.gov/29022676/. https://pubmed.ncbi.nlm.nih.gov/34408425/. https://pubmed.ncbi.nlm.nih.gov/35440329/. https://pubmed.ncbi.nlm.nih.gov/28958142/. https://pubmed.ncbi.nlm.nih.gov/34506449/. https://pubmed.ncbi.nlm.nih.gov/37259407/. https://pubmed.ncbi.nlm.nih.gov/37892562/.

136. Article: https://pubmed.ncbi.nlm.nih.gov/25979770/.

137. Articles: https://pubmed.ncbi.nlm.nih.gov/33852480/.
https://pubmed.ncbi.nlm.nih.gov/30788120/. https://pubmed.ncbi.nlm.nih.gov/35734414/.
138. Articles: https://pubmed.ncbi.nlm.nih.gov/28446599/.
https://pubmed.ncbi.nlm.nih.gov/32535032/. https://pubmed.ncbi.nlm.nih.gov/32252338/.
https://pubmed.ncbi.nlm.nih.gov/34165010/. https://pubmed.ncbi.nlm.nih.gov/36717918/.
https://pubmed.ncbi.nlm.nih.gov/36701289/.
139. Articles: https://pubmed.ncbi.nlm.nih.gov/33183376/.
https://pubmed.ncbi.nlm.nih.gov/35682491/. https://pubmed.ncbi.nlm.nih.gov/36992617/.
https://pubmed.ncbi.nlm.nih.gov/35311615/.
140. Articles: https://www.sciencedaily.com/releases/2021/06/210611174042.htm.
https://www.ncbi.nlm.nih.gov/pmc/articles/PMC8584834/.
https://customcompounding.com.au/new-study-finds-vitamin-d-improves-mental-health-of-those-with
-addictions/.
https://www.alternativetomeds.com/blog/vitamins-addiction-recovery/#:~:text=Co%2Doccurring%
20Disorders%20and%20Vitamin%20Deficiency,-Co%2Doccurring%20psychiatric&text=While%20no
%20pharmaceutical%20has%20been,well%20as%20other%20personality%20disorders.
141. Articles: https://pubmed.ncbi.nlm.nih.gov/33444227/.
https://pubmed.ncbi.nlm.nih.gov/28765037/.
https://pubmed.ncbi.nlm.nih.gov/29522979/.https://pubmed.ncbi.nlm.nih.gov/36313775/.
142. Articles: https://pubmed.ncbi.nlm.nih.gov/36742791/.
https://pubmed.ncbi.nlm.nih.gov/27343963/. https://pubmed.ncbi.nlm.nih.gov/32875143/.
143. Articles: https://pubmed.ncbi.nlm.nih.gov/38853492/.
https://pubmed.ncbi.nlm.nih.gov/35951150/. https://pubmed.ncbi.nlm.nih.gov/38613639/.
144. Article: https://pubmed.ncbi.nlm.nih.gov/29714151/.
145. In my personal experience the condition known as "frozen shoulder" may sometimes be caused by a
vitamin D deficiency. L.S. Articles: https://pubmed.ncbi.nlm.nih.gov/15182797/.
https://www.careatc.com/improving-health/the-link-between-shoulder-pain-and-vitamin-d-deficiency.
https://pubmed.ncbi.nlm.nih.gov/30321335/. https://pubmed.ncbi.nlm.nih.gov/6387576/.
https://pubmed.ncbi.nlm.nih.gov/33390486/. https://pubmed.ncbi.nlm.nih.gov/7014108/.
https://annalsmedres.org/index.php/aomr/article/view/448.
https://www.tampabay.com/news/health/Mayo-Clinic-Q-A-treating-frozen-shoulder-calcium-supple
ments-versus-exercise_165896098/.
https://www.businessinsider.com/guides/health/treatments/frozen-shoulder.
146. Articles: https://pubmed.ncbi.nlm.nih.gov/38966781/.
https://pubmed.ncbi.nlm.nih.gov/37090939/. https://pubmed.ncbi.nlm.nih.gov/36967233/.
147. Articles: https://pubmed.ncbi.nlm.nih.gov/7473848/.
https://pubmed.ncbi.nlm.nih.gov/2880656/. https://pubmed.ncbi.nlm.nih.gov/36137195/.
https://pubmed.ncbi.nlm.nih.gov/33128574/.
148. Related articles: https://pubmed.ncbi.nlm.nih.gov/35268051/.
https://pubmed.ncbi.nlm.nih.gov/35578558/. https://pubmed.ncbi.nlm.nih.gov/32156230/.
149. Article: https://pubmed.ncbi.nlm.nih.gov/28809744/.
150. Article: https://eyesoneyecare.com/resources/ocular-manifestations-vitamin-deficiencies/.
151. Article: https://pubmed.ncbi.nlm.nih.gov/30701762/.
152. Articles: https://pubmed.ncbi.nlm.nih.gov/30078128/.
https://www.ncbi.nlm.nih.gov/pmc/articles/PMC9468237/.
https://www.rupahealth.com/post/an-integrative-medicine-approach-to-agoraphobia-testing-nutrition-
and-evidence-based-therapies.
153. Related article: https://pubmed.ncbi.nlm.nih.gov/33919840/.
154. Article: https://pubmed.ncbi.nlm.nih.gov/30574856/.
https://pubmed.ncbi.nlm.nih.gov/36387030/.
155. Articles: https://pubmed.ncbi.nlm.nih.gov/32099298/.
https://pubmed.ncbi.nlm.nih.gov/1542543/. https://pubmed.ncbi.nlm.nih.gov/19619235/.
https://pubmed.ncbi.nlm.nih.gov/12394373/. https://pubmed.ncbi.nlm.nih.gov/2546510/.
156. Articles: https://pubmed.ncbi.nlm.nih.gov/33183376/.
https://pubmed.ncbi.nlm.nih.gov/28033511/.
157. Articles: https://pubmed.ncbi.nlm.nih.gov/32395409/.
https://pubmed.ncbi.nlm.nih.gov/5365719/.

158. Articles: https://pubmed.ncbi.nlm.nih.gov/36235600/.
https://pubmed.ncbi.nlm.nih.gov/33924232/. https://pubmed.ncbi.nlm.nih.gov/39026686/.
https://pubmed.ncbi.nlm.nih.gov/33435598/. https://pubmed.ncbi.nlm.nih.gov/21872803/.
https://pubmed.ncbi.nlm.nih.gov/20670821/.
159. Articles: https://pubmed.ncbi.nlm.nih.gov/28487837/.
https://pubmed.ncbi.nlm.nih.gov/28102718/. https://pubmed.ncbi.nlm.nih.gov/27188226/.
https://pubmed.ncbi.nlm.nih.gov/34150589/. https://pubmed.ncbi.nlm.nih.gov/37716008/.
160. Article: https://pubmed.ncbi.nlm.nih.gov/31632510/.
161. Article: https://pubmed.ncbi.nlm.nih.gov/24428861/.
162. Article: https://pubmed.ncbi.nlm.nih.gov/23042216/. See also *God-Given Remedies*, p. 163.
163. Articles: https://pubmed.ncbi.nlm.nih.gov/35401868/.
https://pubmed.ncbi.nlm.nih.gov/31310957/. https://pubmed.ncbi.nlm.nih.gov/32550208/.
https://pubmed.ncbi.nlm.nih.gov/28752139/.
164. Article: https://pubmed.ncbi.nlm.nih.gov/24776491/.
165. Articles: https://pubmed.ncbi.nlm.nih.gov/28342017/.
https://pubmed.ncbi.nlm.nih.gov/35800433/. https://pubmed.ncbi.nlm.nih.gov/33710477/.
https://pubmed.ncbi.nlm.nih.gov/36907427/.
166. Article: https://pubmed.ncbi.nlm.nih.gov/24428861/.
167. Articles: https://pubmed.ncbi.nlm.nih.gov/22006065/.
https://pubmed.ncbi.nlm.nih.gov/17606032/. https://pubmed.ncbi.nlm.nih.gov/26803537/.
168. Related articles: https://pubmed.ncbi.nlm.nih.gov/20301602/.
https://pubmed.ncbi.nlm.nih.gov/6289357/.
169. Articles: https://pubmed.ncbi.nlm.nih.gov/38751252/.
https://pubmed.ncbi.nlm.nih.gov/22014374/. https://pubmed.ncbi.nlm.nih.gov/32808447/.
https://pubmed.ncbi.nlm.nih.gov/37108056/. https://pubmed.ncbi.nlm.nih.gov/35449997/.
170. Article: https://www.ncbi.nlm.nih.gov/pmc/articles/PMC4511535/.
171. Article: https://pubmed.ncbi.nlm.nih.gov/27114971/.
172. Articles: https://pubmed.ncbi.nlm.nih.gov/31203645/.
https://pubmed.ncbi.nlm.nih.gov/21322467/. https://pubmed.ncbi.nlm.nih.gov/20406598/.
https://pubmed.ncbi.nlm.nih.gov/36562173/.
173. Article: https://pubmed.ncbi.nlm.nih.gov/36431295/.
174. Article: https://pubmed.ncbi.nlm.nih.gov/25964289/.
175. Article: https://pubmed.ncbi.nlm.nih.gov/25199851/.
176. Articles: https://pubmed.ncbi.nlm.nih.gov/25445242/.
https://pubmed.ncbi.nlm.nih.gov/37919813/. https://pubmed.ncbi.nlm.nih.gov/30959831/.
177. Articles: https://pubmed.ncbi.nlm.nih.gov/29126718/.
https://pubmed.ncbi.nlm.nih.gov/30282560/. https://pubmed.ncbi.nlm.nih.gov/38534213/.
https://pubmed.ncbi.nlm.nih.gov/22635218/. https://pubmed.ncbi.nlm.nih.gov/27994369/.
178. Articles: https://pubmed.ncbi.nlm.nih.gov/2736265/.
https://www.cambridge.org/core/journals/psychological-medicine/article/abs/vitamin-d-sufficiency-a
ttenuates-the-effect-of-early-social-adversity-on-child-antisocial-behavior/5931BD4BF05EFF5266557FC
279F4A2EF.
179. Articles: https://pubmed.ncbi.nlm.nih.gov/26680471/.
https://www.ncbi.nlm.nih.gov/pmc/articles/PMC4511535/
180. Articles: https://pubmed.ncbi.nlm.nih.gov/34518086/.
https://pubmed.ncbi.nlm.nih.gov/26603433/. https://pubmed.ncbi.nlm.nih.gov/33797793/.
https://pubmed.ncbi.nlm.nih.gov/29400142/. https://pubmed.ncbi.nlm.nih.gov/32936248/.
https://pubmed.ncbi.nlm.nih.gov/22841360/.
181. Articles: https://pubmed.ncbi.nlm.nih.gov/31493304/.
https://pubmed.ncbi.nlm.nih.gov/37426194/. https://pubmed.ncbi.nlm.nih.gov/28786261/.
182. Article: https://www.lybrate.com/topic/appendicitis-diet.
183. Article: https://pubmed.ncbi.nlm.nih.gov/35198590/.
184. Articles: https://pubmed.ncbi.nlm.nih.gov/29126718/.
https://pubmed.ncbi.nlm.nih.gov/30282560/. https://pubmed.ncbi.nlm.nih.gov/38534213/.
https://pubmed.ncbi.nlm.nih.gov/22635218/. https://pubmed.ncbi.nlm.nih.gov/27994369/.

185. Articles: https://pubmed.ncbi.nlm.nih.gov/28446599/.
https://pubmed.ncbi.nlm.nih.gov/32535032/. https://pubmed.ncbi.nlm.nih.gov/32252338/.
https://pubmed.ncbi.nlm.nih.gov/34165010/. https://pubmed.ncbi.nlm.nih.gov/36717918/.
https://pubmed.ncbi.nlm.nih.gov/36701289/.
186. Related article: https://www.ncbi.nlm.nih.gov/pmc/articles/PMC9220304/.
187. Articles: https://pubmed.ncbi.nlm.nih.gov/22841360/.
https://pubmed.ncbi.nlm.nih.gov/23703334/. https://pubmed.ncbi.nlm.nih.gov/32520144/.
https://pubmed.ncbi.nlm.nih.gov/24436433/.
188. Articles: https://pubmed.ncbi.nlm.nih.gov/33485122/.
https://pubmed.ncbi.nlm.nih.gov/35834511/. https://pubmed.ncbi.nlm.nih.gov/31653092/.
189. Article: https://pubmed.ncbi.nlm.nih.gov/31286174/.
190. Articles: https://pubmed.ncbi.nlm.nih.gov/33724323/.
https://pubmed.ncbi.nlm.nih.gov/35451180/. https://pubmed.ncbi.nlm.nih.gov/25705008/.
https://pubmed.ncbi.nlm.nih.gov/29154815/. https://pubmed.ncbi.nlm.nih.gov/27556176/.
191. Articles: https://pubmed.ncbi.nlm.nih.gov/32294031/.
https://pubmed.ncbi.nlm.nih.gov/33383952/. https://pubmed.ncbi.nlm.nih.gov/31755381/.
https://pubmed.ncbi.nlm.nih.gov/34602240/.
192. Articles:
https://www.frontiersin.org/journals/behavioral-neuroscience/articles/10.3389/fnbeh.2022.859151/
full. https://www.ncbi.nlm.nih.gov/pmc/articles/PMC9128593/.
https://www.ncbi.nlm.nih.gov/pmc/articles/PMC4302541/.
193. Articles: https://pubmed.ncbi.nlm.nih.gov/33019741/.
https://pubmed.ncbi.nlm.nih.gov/25231772/. https://pubmed.ncbi.nlm.nih.gov/29314357/.
https://pubmed.ncbi.nlm.nih.gov/32485309/. https://pubmed.ncbi.nlm.nih.gov/27011794/.
194. Article: https://pubmed.ncbi.nlm.nih.gov/36744416/.
195. Article: https://pubmed.ncbi.nlm.nih.gov/31377030/.
196. Article: https://pubmed.ncbi.nlm.nih.gov/36943351/.
197. Article: https://www.healthline.com/nutrition/vitamin-d-deficiency-symptoms.
198. Article: https://pubmed.ncbi.nlm.nih.gov/32245151/. See also Ryan, pp. 51-55.
199. Articles: https://pubmed.ncbi.nlm.nih.gov/27918470/.
https://pubmed.ncbi.nlm.nih.gov/32419030/. https://pubmed.ncbi.nlm.nih.gov/36558443/.
https://pubmed.ncbi.nlm.nih.gov/25985948/. https://pubmed.ncbi.nlm.nih.gov/31405041/.
https://pubmed.ncbi.nlm.nih.gov/25973433/. https://pubmed.ncbi.nlm.nih.gov/27061361/.
200. Articles: https://pubmed.ncbi.nlm.nih.gov/35763390/.
https://pubmed.ncbi.nlm.nih.gov/26239464/. https://pubmed.ncbi.nlm.nih.gov/31405041/.
https://pubmed.ncbi.nlm.nih.gov/33145984/.
201. Articles: https://pubmed.ncbi.nlm.nih.gov/33724323/.
https://pubmed.ncbi.nlm.nih.gov/35451180/. https://pubmed.ncbi.nlm.nih.gov/37236436/.
https://pubmed.ncbi.nlm.nih.gov/37375629/. https://pubmed.ncbi.nlm.nih.gov/31727055/.
202. Related articles: https://pubmed.ncbi.nlm.nih.gov/6185056/.
https://pubmed.ncbi.nlm.nih.gov/18795911/. https://pubmed.ncbi.nlm.nih.gov/4244469/.
203. Article: https://pubmed.ncbi.nlm.nih.gov/33865361/.
204. Article: https://pubmed.ncbi.nlm.nih.gov/29714151/.
205. Article: https://pubmed.ncbi.nlm.nih.gov/32294031/.
206. Articles: https://pubmed.ncbi.nlm.nih.gov/32294031/.
https://pubmed.ncbi.nlm.nih.gov/33383952/. https://pubmed.ncbi.nlm.nih.gov/31755381/.
https://pubmed.ncbi.nlm.nih.gov/34602240/.
207. Related articles: https://pubmed.ncbi.nlm.nih.gov/32200644/.
https://pubmed.ncbi.nlm.nih.gov/35535019/.
208. Articles: https://pubmed.ncbi.nlm.nih.gov/36231195/.
https://www.webmd.com/vitamins-and-supplements/what-to-know-about-vitamin-d-and-mental-healt
h.
209. Articles: https://pubmed.ncbi.nlm.nih.gov/28315909/.
https://pubmed.ncbi.nlm.nih.gov/38542128/. https://pubmed.ncbi.nlm.nih.gov/33679732/.
https://pubmed.ncbi.nlm.nih.gov/36501065/.
210. Articles: https://pubmed.ncbi.nlm.nih.gov/31038320/.
https://pubmed.ncbi.nlm.nih.gov/15223208/.
211. Article: https://pubmed.ncbi.nlm.nih.gov/36212121/. See also Altshul and Hops, p. 164; Holick,
p. 68.

212. Article: https://pubmed.ncbi.nlm.nih.gov/35198149/.
213. Articles: https://pubmed.ncbi.nlm.nih.gov/37024856/.
https://pubmed.ncbi.nlm.nih.gov/36483925/. https://pubmed.ncbi.nlm.nih.gov/22900656/.
https://pubmed.ncbi.nlm.nih.gov/31304052/. https://pubmed.ncbi.nlm.nih.gov/24722382/.
214. Articles: https://pubmed.ncbi.nlm.nih.gov/26156834/.
https://pubmed.ncbi.nlm.nih.gov/26800885/. https://pubmed.ncbi.nlm.nih.gov/35076925/.
https://pubmed.ncbi.nlm.nih.gov/31660939/.
215. Articles: https://pubmed.ncbi.nlm.nih.gov/20956641/.
https://pubmed.ncbi.nlm.nih.gov/15088627/. https://pubmed.ncbi.nlm.nih.gov/17204418/.
216. Article: https://pubmed.ncbi.nlm.nih.gov/28273374/.
217. Related articles: https://www.ncbi.nlm.nih.gov/pmc/articles/PMC9974688/.
https://pubmed.ncbi.nlm.nih.gov/37011375/.
218. Article: https://maze.conductscience.com/vitamin-d-and-anxiety/.
219. Articles: https://pubmed.ncbi.nlm.nih.gov/36655442/.
https://pubmed.ncbi.nlm.nih.gov/35184713/. https://pubmed.ncbi.nlm.nih.gov/32593521/.
https://pubmed.ncbi.nlm.nih.gov/30789802/.
220. Articles:
https://www.asbestos.com/treatment/nutrition/cancer-fighting-vitamins/#:~:text=A%202021%20cl
inical%20research%20study,Healthy%20foods%20containing%20vitamin%20D.
221. Articles: https://pubmed.ncbi.nlm.nih.gov/33231724/.
https://pubmed.ncbi.nlm.nih.gov/32759193/. https://pubmed.ncbi.nlm.nih.gov/32839838/.
https://pubmed.ncbi.nlm.nih.gov/35878631/. https://pubmed.ncbi.nlm.nih.gov/35747111/.
https://pubmed.ncbi.nlm.nih.gov/35418365/. https://pubmed.ncbi.nlm.nih.gov/37807761/.
222. Articles: https://pubmed.ncbi.nlm.nih.gov/31451276/.
https://pubmed.ncbi.nlm.nih.gov/36714231/. https://pubmed.ncbi.nlm.nih.gov/27327576/.
https://pubmed.ncbi.nlm.nih.gov/24979517/. https://pubmed.ncbi.nlm.nih.gov/25864760/.
223. Article: https://pubmed.ncbi.nlm.nih.gov/22991390/.
224. Articles: https://pubmed.ncbi.nlm.nih.gov/27876139/.
https://pubmed.ncbi.nlm.nih.gov/18211975/. https://pubmed.ncbi.nlm.nih.gov/25070319/.
https://pubmed.ncbi.nlm.nih.gov/32467771/. https://pubmed.ncbi.nlm.nih.gov/38633760/.
225. Articles: https://pubmed.ncbi.nlm.nih.gov/33626532/.
https://pubmed.ncbi.nlm.nih.gov/28256614/. https://pubmed.ncbi.nlm.nih.gov/24939880/.
https://pubmed.ncbi.nlm.nih.gov/23375797/.
226. Articles: https://pubmed.ncbi.nlm.nih.gov/25130505/.
https://pubmed.ncbi.nlm.nih.gov/38772131/.
https://neomesia.com/assets/files/approfondimenti/Todisco-Relation-between-vitamin-D-and-impulse
-behaviours-in-patients-with-eating-disorder-a-pilot-observational-study.pdf.
227. Article: https://pubmed.ncbi.nlm.nih.gov/25713056/.
228. Articles: https://pubmed.ncbi.nlm.nih.gov/37321901/.
https://pubmed.ncbi.nlm.nih.gov/36370297/. https://pubmed.ncbi.nlm.nih.gov/34080787/.
https://pubmed.ncbi.nlm.nih.gov/30972950/. https://pubmed.ncbi.nlm.nih.gov/20978193/.
229. Article: https://pubmed.ncbi.nlm.nih.gov/31930458/.
230. Articles: https://pubmed.ncbi.nlm.nih.gov/31722876/.
https://pubmed.ncbi.nlm.nih.gov/35684153/. https://pubmed.ncbi.nlm.nih.gov/35673423/.
https://pubmed.ncbi.nlm.nih.gov/28858875/.
231. Article: https://pubmed.ncbi.nlm.nih.gov/36890539/.
232. Article:
https://www.verywellhealth.com/vitamin-d-may-help-some-cancer-therapies-work-2252049.
233. Article: https://pubmed.ncbi.nlm.nih.gov/31402402/.
234. Articles: https://pubmed.ncbi.nlm.nih.gov/27276637/.
https://pubmed.ncbi.nlm.nih.gov/21102216/. https://pubmed.ncbi.nlm.nih.gov/34209445/.
235. Articles: https://pubmed.ncbi.nlm.nih.gov/28436021/.
https://pubmed.ncbi.nlm.nih.gov/37810154/. https://pubmed.ncbi.nlm.nih.gov/38390354/.
https://pubmed.ncbi.nlm.nih.gov/38920853/.
236. Article: https://pubmed.ncbi.nlm.nih.gov/37378487/.
237. Related articles: https://www.ncbi.nlm.nih.gov/pmc/articles/PMC9974688/.
https://pubmed.ncbi.nlm.nih.gov/37011375/.
238. Related articles: https://www.ncbi.nlm.nih.gov/pmc/articles/PMC4802895/.
https://jamanetwork.com/journals/jamanetworkopen/fullarticle/2787456.

239. Articles: https://pubmed.ncbi.nlm.nih.gov/29657326/.
https://pubmed.ncbi.nlm.nih.gov/18460265/. https://pubmed.ncbi.nlm.nih.gov/15585788/.
https://pubmed.ncbi.nlm.nih.gov/22461123/. https://pubmed.ncbi.nlm.nih.gov/29951549/.
240. Article: https://pubmed.ncbi.nlm.nih.gov/34284830/.
241. Related articles: https://pubmed.ncbi.nlm.nih.gov/31068690/.
https://pubmed.ncbi.nlm.nih.gov/29435763/. https://pubmed.ncbi.nlm.nih.gov/30253289/.
https://pubmed.ncbi.nlm.nih.gov/31233632/. https://pubmed.ncbi.nlm.nih.gov/38777417/.
242. See "Diet, Nutrition and the Prevention of Osteoporosis," Cambridge University Press. Article:
https://www.cambridge.org/core/journals/public-health-nutrition/article/diet-nutrition-and-the-prev
ention-of-osteoporosis/70C8DDD13DEF94A9AFE89F3F93E1A097.
243. Article: https://pubmed.ncbi.nlm.nih.gov/29931664/. See also Weiss, p. 157.
244. Articles: https://pubmed.ncbi.nlm.nih.gov/18088161/.
https://pubmed.ncbi.nlm.nih.gov/18460265/. https://pubmed.ncbi.nlm.nih.gov/18400738/.
https://pubmed.ncbi.nlm.nih.gov/24119980/. https://pubmed.ncbi.nlm.nih.gov/30321335/.
https://pubmed.ncbi.nlm.nih.gov/31860103/. https://pubmed.ncbi.nlm.nih.gov/32785003/. See
also Holick, pp. 198-202.
245. Article: https://pubmed.ncbi.nlm.nih.gov/24119980/.
246. Article: https://pubmed.ncbi.nlm.nih.gov/21193656/.
247. Article: https://pubmed.ncbi.nlm.nih.gov/31239976/.
248. Article: https://pubmed.ncbi.nlm.nih.gov/21872800/.
249. Articles: https://pubmed.ncbi.nlm.nih.gov/21486172/. https://foodforthebrain.org/bpd/.
https://www.hopeforbpd.com/borderline-personality-disorder-treatment/treating-borderline-personal
ity-disorder-without-drugs.
https://www.amenclinics.com/blog/what-you-dont-know-about-borderline-personality-disorder/.
https://www.nutritank.com/borderline-personality-disorder-and-nutrition.
250. Article: https://pubmed.ncbi.nlm.nih.gov/13413694/.
251. Articles: https://pubmed.ncbi.nlm.nih.gov/26811638/.
https://pubmed.ncbi.nlm.nih.gov/37530744/. https://pubmed.ncbi.nlm.nih.gov/36946647/.
https://pubmed.ncbi.nlm.nih.gov/21801808/.
252. See also fecal incontinence. Articles: https://pubmed.ncbi.nlm.nih.gov/24807423/.
https://pubmed.ncbi.nlm.nih.gov/38316640/. https://pubmed.ncbi.nlm.nih.gov/20232146/.
253. Articles: https://pubmed.ncbi.nlm.nih.gov/15671222/.
https://pubmed.ncbi.nlm.nih.gov/16353199/. https://pubmed.ncbi.nlm.nih.gov/16214919/.
254. Articles: https://pubmed.ncbi.nlm.nih.gov/33231724/.
https://pubmed.ncbi.nlm.nih.gov/32759193/. https://pubmed.ncbi.nlm.nih.gov/32839838/.
https://pubmed.ncbi.nlm.nih.gov/35878631/. https://pubmed.ncbi.nlm.nih.gov/35747111/.
https://pubmed.ncbi.nlm.nih.gov/35418365/. https://pubmed.ncbi.nlm.nih.gov/37807761/.
255. Articles: https://pubmed.ncbi.nlm.nih.gov/38241458/.
https://pubmed.ncbi.nlm.nih.gov/36034296/. https://pubmed.ncbi.nlm.nih.gov/33145201/.
https://pubmed.ncbi.nlm.nih.gov/34088910/. https://pubmed.ncbi.nlm.nih.gov/38347057/.
https://pubmed.ncbi.nlm.nih.gov/36764983/.
256. Article: https://pubmed.ncbi.nlm.nih.gov/34642910/.
257. Article: https://onlinelibrary.wiley.com/doi/full/10.1002/cns3.4.
258. Articles: https://www.ncbi.nlm.nih.gov/pmc/articles/PMC6132681/.
https://www.medicalnewstoday.com/articles/283971.
https://pubmed.ncbi.nlm.nih.gov/33562339/. https://pubmed.ncbi.nlm.nih.gov/19019042/.
https://pubmed.ncbi.nlm.nih.gov/12853323/.
259. Articles: https://pubmed.ncbi.nlm.nih.gov/38846332/.
https://pubmed.ncbi.nlm.nih.gov/31181357/. https://pubmed.ncbi.nlm.nih.gov/25348494/.
https://pubmed.ncbi.nlm.nih.gov/34504307/.
260. *Food and Nutrition*, p. 30; Khalsa, pp. 82-88; Holick, pp. 80-81; Zaidi, pp. 106-114. See also
articles: https://pubmed.ncbi.nlm.nih.gov/23042216/.
https://pubmed.ncbi.nlm.nih.gov/30041759/.
261. Article: https://pubmed.ncbi.nlm.nih.gov/18460265/.
262. Articles: https://pubmed.ncbi.nlm.nih.gov/28828295/.
https://pubmed.ncbi.nlm.nih.gov/30827468/. https://pubmed.ncbi.nlm.nih.gov/29490469/.
https://pubmed.ncbi.nlm.nih.gov/23076388/.
263. Article: https://pubmed.ncbi.nlm.nih.gov/32647146/.

264. Articles: https://pubmed.ncbi.nlm.nih.gov/33878208/.
https://pubmed.ncbi.nlm.nih.gov/30246004/. https://pubmed.ncbi.nlm.nih.gov/35049200/.
https://pubmed.ncbi.nlm.nih.gov/32628705/. https://pubmed.ncbi.nlm.nih.gov/33878218/.
https://pubmed.ncbi.nlm.nih.gov/27467562/. https://pubmed.ncbi.nlm.nih.gov/34989171/.
265. Related articles:
https://assets.ctfassets.net/e0h7lzmer4zr/FOh1r2W6CO02kbjEl1aoE/e1bc49fe9f5ea8707c5f50aca9b2
f7b2/ICMCRJ-3-1418.pdf. https://www.pagepress.org/journals/index.php/dr/article/view/9418.
https://www.pagepress.org/journals/dr/article/view/9705.
266. Articles: https://pubmed.ncbi.nlm.nih.gov/34540161/.
https://pubmed.ncbi.nlm.nih.gov/36542233/. https://pubmed.ncbi.nlm.nih.gov/26927460/.
https://pubmed.ncbi.nlm.nih.gov/31940296/.
267. Articles: https://pubmed.ncbi.nlm.nih.gov/23276942/.
https://pubmed.ncbi.nlm.nih.gov/20954138/.
268. Articles: https://pubmed.ncbi.nlm.nih.gov/33413308/.
https://pubmed.ncbi.nlm.nih.gov/35128822/. https://pubmed.ncbi.nlm.nih.gov/37869762/.
https://pubmed.ncbi.nlm.nih.gov/36226108/.
269. Related articles: https://pubmed.ncbi.nlm.nih.gov/37732453/.
https://pubmed.ncbi.nlm.nih.gov/32771307/.
270. Articles: https://pubmed.ncbi.nlm.nih.gov/7565066/.
https://pubmed.ncbi.nlm.nih.gov/10475815/. https://pubmed.ncbi.nlm.nih.gov/38772131/.
271. Article: https://www.ncbi.nlm.nih.gov/pmc/articles/PMC4511535/.
272. Articles: https://pubmed.ncbi.nlm.nih.gov/30343406/.
https://www.anklefootmd.com/vitamin-d-can-boost-healing-following-bunion-surgery/.
https://www.bunionsurgeryspecialistsllc.com/vitamin-and-mineral-supplementation-for-bone-health/.
273. Articles: https://pubmed.ncbi.nlm.nih.gov/28436021/.
https://pubmed.ncbi.nlm.nih.gov/37810154/. https://pubmed.ncbi.nlm.nih.gov/38390354/.
https://pubmed.ncbi.nlm.nih.gov/38920853/.
274. Articles: https://pubmed.ncbi.nlm.nih.gov/22367532/.
https://pubmed.ncbi.nlm.nih.gov/22332088/. https://pubmed.ncbi.nlm.nih.gov/29776863/.
https://pubmed.ncbi.nlm.nih.gov/24011706/.
275. Articles: https://pubmed.ncbi.nlm.nih.gov/33590380/.
https://pubmed.ncbi.nlm.nih.gov/38348080/. https://pubmed.ncbi.nlm.nih.gov/37943388/.
https://pubmed.ncbi.nlm.nih.gov/27499590/. https://pubmed.ncbi.nlm.nih.gov/31905893/.
https://pubmed.ncbi.nlm.nih.gov/35546270/. https://pubmed.ncbi.nlm.nih.gov/30858945/.
276. Article: https://pubmed.ncbi.nlm.nih.gov/34981132/.
277. Articles: https://pubmed.ncbi.nlm.nih.gov/25960299/.
https://pubmed.ncbi.nlm.nih.gov/37809218/. https://pubmed.ncbi.nlm.nih.gov/29523679/.
https://pubmed.ncbi.nlm.nih.gov/27566435/. https://pubmed.ncbi.nlm.nih.gov/28212442/.
https://pubmed.ncbi.nlm.nih.gov/30304522/.
278. Related article: https://pubmed.ncbi.nlm.nih.gov/16121806/.
279. Articles: https://pubmed.ncbi.nlm.nih.gov/27865660/.
https://pubmed.ncbi.nlm.nih.gov/30773722/. https://pubmed.ncbi.nlm.nih.gov/36162148/.
https://pubmed.ncbi.nlm.nih.gov/30193921/. https://pubmed.ncbi.nlm.nih.gov/27321391/.
280. Articles: https://pubmed.ncbi.nlm.nih.gov/26860322/.
https://pubmed.ncbi.nlm.nih.gov/38375518/. https://pubmed.ncbi.nlm.nih.gov/38373939/.
https://pubmed.ncbi.nlm.nih.gov/22538413/. https://pubmed.ncbi.nlm.nih.gov/33096916/.
https://pubmed.ncbi.nlm.nih.gov/25612733/. https://pubmed.ncbi.nlm.nih.gov/36162148/.
281. Article: https://www.ncbi.nlm.nih.gov/pmc/articles/PMC6230238/.
https://www.ijpsonline.com/articles/impact-of-vitamin-dsub3sub-supplementation-on-recurrent-aphth
ous-ulcer-4515.html.
282. Articles: https://pubmed.ncbi.nlm.nih.gov/30878964/.
https://pubmed.ncbi.nlm.nih.gov/192079/.
283. Articles: https://pubmed.ncbi.nlm.nih.gov/27026421/.
https://pubmed.ncbi.nlm.nih.gov/30878964/. https://pubmed.ncbi.nlm.nih.gov/34095466/.
https://pubmed.ncbi.nlm.nih.gov/22493603/.
284. Article: https://pubmed.ncbi.nlm.nih.gov/30415629/. See also Ryan, pp. 81-85.

285. Articles: https://pubmed.ncbi.nlm.nih.gov/34490545/.
https://pubmed.ncbi.nlm.nih.gov/37151171/. https://pubmed.ncbi.nlm.nih.gov/32765854/.
https://pubmed.ncbi.nlm.nih.gov/32294751/. https://pubmed.ncbi.nlm.nih.gov/27062466/.
https://pubmed.ncbi.nlm.nih.gov/26701973/. https://pubmed.ncbi.nlm.nih.gov/28552837/.
https://pubmed.ncbi.nlm.nih.gov/33472438/.
286. Article: https://pubmed.ncbi.nlm.nih.gov/21633708/.
287. Articles: https://pubmed.ncbi.nlm.nih.gov/35457041/.
https://pubmed.ncbi.nlm.nih.gov/38214845/. https://pubmed.ncbi.nlm.nih.gov/32575105/.
https://pubmed.ncbi.nlm.nih.gov/36174848/. https://pubmed.ncbi.nlm.nih.gov/33029234/.
https://pubmed.ncbi.nlm.nih.gov/26124632/.
288. Articles: https://pubmed.ncbi.nlm.nih.gov/19687184/.
https://pubmed.ncbi.nlm.nih.gov/37339367/. https://pubmed.ncbi.nlm.nih.gov/34095485/.
289. Articles: https://www.ncbi.nlm.nih.gov/pmc/articles/PMC9220304/.
https://www.ahajournals.org/doi/10.1161/RES.0000000000000229.
290. Articles: https://pubmed.ncbi.nlm.nih.gov/34064075/.
https://pubmed.ncbi.nlm.nih.gov/36916243/. https://pubmed.ncbi.nlm.nih.gov/36927535/.
https://pubmed.ncbi.nlm.nih.gov/27930380/.
291. Articles: https://pubmed.ncbi.nlm.nih.gov/35531196/.
https://pubmed.ncbi.nlm.nih.gov/36031913/. https://pubmed.ncbi.nlm.nih.gov/29342407/.
https://pubmed.ncbi.nlm.nih.gov/34371988/. https://pubmed.ncbi.nlm.nih.gov/35023113/.
https://pubmed.ncbi.nlm.nih.gov/18058622/.
292. Article: https://pubmed.ncbi.nlm.nih.gov/36678205/.
293. Articles: https://pubmed.ncbi.nlm.nih.gov/24746456/.
https://pubmed.ncbi.nlm.nih.gov/28786261/. https://pubmed.ncbi.nlm.nih.gov/30870794/.
294. Articles: https://pubmed.ncbi.nlm.nih.gov/38230221/.
https://pubmed.ncbi.nlm.nih.gov/37240017/. https://pubmed.ncbi.nlm.nih.gov/33112551/.
https://pubmed.ncbi.nlm.nih.gov/38913397/. https://pubmed.ncbi.nlm.nih.gov/29113037/.
295. Articles: https://pubmed.ncbi.nlm.nih.gov/27588820/.
https://pubmed.ncbi.nlm.nih.gov/20144597/. https://pubmed.ncbi.nlm.nih.gov/30848027/.
296. Article: https://pubmed.ncbi.nlm.nih.gov/35565867/. One study showed that pregnant vitamin D deficient women were more likely to require a C-section. See Zaidi, p. 165.
297. Article: https://pubmed.ncbi.nlm.nih.gov/20209476/.
298. Article: https://cancercenterforhealing.com/dry-lips-vitamin-deficiency/.
299. Article: https://cancercenterforhealing.com/dry-lips-vitamin-deficiency/.
300. Articles: https://pubmed.ncbi.nlm.nih.gov/31949283/.
https://pubmed.ncbi.nlm.nih.gov/36866055/.
301. Articles: https://pubmed.ncbi.nlm.nih.gov/35458189/.
https://pubmed.ncbi.nlm.nih.gov/35352542/. https://pubmed.ncbi.nlm.nih.gov/28923762/.
302. Article: https://pubmed.ncbi.nlm.nih.gov/30588571/.
303. Articles: https://www.healthylife.com.au/learn/chicken-pox.
https://pubmed.ncbi.nlm.nih.gov/25487609/. https://pubmed.ncbi.nlm.nih.gov/38423817/.
https://www.ukbiobank.ac.uk/enable-your-research/approved-research/association-between-serum-vi tamin-d-deficiency-and-the-risk-of-herpes-zoster-a-longitudinal-uk-biobank-study.
304. Articles: https://pubmed.ncbi.nlm.nih.gov/18933785/.
https://pubmed.ncbi.nlm.nih.gov/33653127/. https://pubmed.ncbi.nlm.nih.gov/4974562/.
305. Articles: https://pubmed.ncbi.nlm.nih.gov/38698906/.
https://pubmed.ncbi.nlm.nih.gov/23201171/.
306. Articles: https://pubmed.ncbi.nlm.nih.gov/33626532/.
https://pubmed.ncbi.nlm.nih.gov/28256614/. https://pubmed.ncbi.nlm.nih.gov/24939880/.
https://pubmed.ncbi.nlm.nih.gov/23375797/.
307. Articles: https://pubmed.ncbi.nlm.nih.gov/36605198/.
https://pubmed.ncbi.nlm.nih.gov/33021858/. https://pubmed.ncbi.nlm.nih.gov/36771282/.
https://pubmed.ncbi.nlm.nih.gov/35215528/. https://pubmed.ncbi.nlm.nih.gov/23845396/.
308. Articles: https://pubmed.ncbi.nlm.nih.gov/38529069/.
https://pubmed.ncbi.nlm.nih.gov/12455400/. https://pubmed.ncbi.nlm.nih.gov/8148393/.
https://pubmed.ncbi.nlm.nih.gov/34137176/.
309. Articles: https://pubmed.ncbi.nlm.nih.gov/29715698/.
https://pubmed.ncbi.nlm.nih.gov/33170652/. https://pubmed.ncbi.nlm.nih.gov/32270179/.
https://pubmed.ncbi.nlm.nih.gov/35533917/. https://pubmed.ncbi.nlm.nih.gov/28514918/.

310. Article: https://pubmed.ncbi.nlm.nih.gov/36627071/.

311. Articles: https://pubmed.ncbi.nlm.nih.gov/36013312/.
https://pubmed.ncbi.nlm.nih.gov/37892562/. https://pubmed.ncbi.nlm.nih.gov/27499590/.
Related article: https://pubmed.ncbi.nlm.nih.gov/26889405/.

312. Article: https://pubmed.ncbi.nlm.nih.gov/29118054/.

313. Articles: https://pubmed.ncbi.nlm.nih.gov/21048153/.
https://pubmed.ncbi.nlm.nih.gov/33466695/. https://pubmed.ncbi.nlm.nih.gov/38701347/.
https://pubmed.ncbi.nlm.nih.gov/22047708/. https://pubmed.ncbi.nlm.nih.gov/27333923/.
https://pubmed.ncbi.nlm.nih.gov/28157213/. https://pubmed.ncbi.nlm.nih.gov/21883139/.

314. Articles: https://pubmed.ncbi.nlm.nih.gov/37643857/.
https://pubmed.ncbi.nlm.nih.gov/37880985/. https://pubmed.ncbi.nlm.nih.gov/30255465/.
https://pubmed.ncbi.nlm.nih.gov/8635507/.

315. Article: https://pubmed.ncbi.nlm.nih.gov/36562273/.

316. Article: https://www.ncbi.nlm.nih.gov/pmc/articles/PMC4170888/.

317. Articles: https://pubmed.ncbi.nlm.nih.gov/35734414/.
https://pubmed.ncbi.nlm.nih.gov/28029611/. https://pubmed.ncbi.nlm.nih.gov/38989753/.
https://pubmed.ncbi.nlm.nih.gov/31558406/.

318. Articles: https://pubmed.ncbi.nlm.nih.gov/33129807/.
https://pubmed.ncbi.nlm.nih.gov/38089624/. https://pubmed.ncbi.nlm.nih.gov/37661839/.
https://pubmed.ncbi.nlm.nih.gov/38999859/. https://pubmed.ncbi.nlm.nih.gov/30843734/.
https://pubmed.ncbi.nlm.nih.gov/28353643/.

319. Articles: https://pubmed.ncbi.nlm.nih.gov/36142636/.
https://pubmed.ncbi.nlm.nih.gov/34774723/. https://pubmed.ncbi.nlm.nih.gov/37815065/.
https://pubmed.ncbi.nlm.nih.gov/31789949/. https://pubmed.ncbi.nlm.nih.gov/22113744/.
https://pubmed.ncbi.nlm.nih.gov/37155562/.

320. Article: https://www.dshs.texas.gov/citrullinemia.

321. Article: https://pubmed.ncbi.nlm.nih.gov/23843449/.

322. There is growing evidence that a vitamin D deficiency can cause cluster headaches. Thus some studies also show that vitamin D can prevent, slow, and/or reduce the pain and number of attacks; meaning that it can be used as both a preventative and a treatment. See articles:
https://pubmed.ncbi.nlm.nih.gov/30019090/. https://pubmed.ncbi.nlm.nih.gov/37539938/.
https://pubmed.ncbi.nlm.nih.gov/36983024/.

323. Articles: https://pubmed.ncbi.nlm.nih.gov/25623479/.
https://pubmed.ncbi.nlm.nih.gov/34989311/. https://pubmed.ncbi.nlm.nih.gov/24492311/.
https://pubmed.ncbi.nlm.nih.gov/25479065/. https://pubmed.ncbi.nlm.nih.gov/37416010/.
https://pubmed.ncbi.nlm.nih.gov/25471926/.

324. Articles: https://pubmed.ncbi.nlm.nih.gov/21295360/.
https://pubmed.ncbi.nlm.nih.gov/24265555/. https://pubmed.ncbi.nlm.nih.gov/2204648/.

325. Articles: https://pubmed.ncbi.nlm.nih.gov/3927224/.
https://pubmed.ncbi.nlm.nih.gov/6602194/. https://pubmed.ncbi.nlm.nih.gov/10205935/.
https://pubmed.ncbi.nlm.nih.gov/6712083/. https://pubmed.ncbi.nlm.nih.gov/3976850/.

326. Articles: https://pubmed.ncbi.nlm.nih.gov/34064075/.
https://pubmed.ncbi.nlm.nih.gov/36916243/. https://pubmed.ncbi.nlm.nih.gov/36927535/.
https://pubmed.ncbi.nlm.nih.gov/27930380/.

327. Article: https://pubmed.ncbi.nlm.nih.gov/34981132/.

328. Article: https://pubmed.ncbi.nlm.nih.gov/30795846/.

329. Articles: https://pubmed.ncbi.nlm.nih.gov/36636389/.
https://pubmed.ncbi.nlm.nih.gov/31145049/. https://pubmed.ncbi.nlm.nih.gov/37081493/.

330. Article: https://pubmed.ncbi.nlm.nih.gov/35236213/.

331. Article: https://pubmed.ncbi.nlm.nih.gov/37478851/. Because it can suppress the growth of cancer cells, vitamin D has been found to be successful in both preventing and treating a myriad of cancers. *Food and Nutrition*, p. 30; see also Zaidi, pp. 106-114; Khalsa, pp. 92-94.

332. Articles: https://pubmed.ncbi.nlm.nih.gov/33058307/.
https://pubmed.ncbi.nlm.nih.gov/27768599/. https://pubmed.ncbi.nlm.nih.gov/31837045/.

333. Articles: https://pubmed.ncbi.nlm.nih.gov/36282253/.
https://pubmed.ncbi.nlm.nih.gov/31086686/. https://pubmed.ncbi.nlm.nih.gov/33237839/.
https://pubmed.ncbi.nlm.nih.gov/32882734/. https://pubmed.ncbi.nlm.nih.gov/29501468/.

334. Article: https://pubmed.ncbi.nlm.nih.gov/23032554/. Taking 5,000 IU of vitamin D daily has been shown to keep the body strong and reduce the risk of getting sick. *Bottom Line's 2021 Health Breakthroughs*, p. 249.

335. Article: https://pubmed.ncbi.nlm.nih.gov/32795337/.

336. Articles:
https://pubmed.ncbi.nlm.nih.gov/31518608/#:~:text=population%2Dbased%20sample-,Posttrauma tic%20stress%20disorder%20is%20associated%20with%20reduced%20vitamin%20D%20levels,Jan%20 10%3A96%3A109760.
https://www.psychiatrictimes.com/view/exploring-integrative-medicine-and-nutrition-for-ptsd.
https://foodforthebrain.org/ptsd/.

337. Related articles:
https://thedawnrehab.com/blog/12-supplements-that-benefit-recovery-from-addiction/.
https://www.paracelsus-recovery.com/blog/vitamin-d-and-addiction/.

338. Article:
https://www.webmd.com/vitamins-and-supplements/what-to-know-about-vitamin-d-and-mental-healt h.

339. Related articles:
https://sph.umich.edu/news/2019posts/low-levels-vitamin-d-elementary-school-could-spell-trouble-in -adolescence.html#:~:text=New%20Research%20from%20Eduardo%20Villamor&text=Children%20 with%20blood%20vitamin%20D,higher%20levels%20of%20the%20vitamin.
https://www.ncbi.nlm.nih.gov/pmc/articles/PMC7011463/.

340. Articles: https://pubmed.ncbi.nlm.nih.gov/33550671/.
https://pubmed.ncbi.nlm.nih.gov/27730031/. https://pubmed.ncbi.nlm.nih.gov/33764502/.

341. Article: https://www.ncbi.nlm.nih.gov/pmc/articles/PMC4511535/.

342. Related article: https://pubmed.ncbi.nlm.nih.gov/37869762/.

343. Articles: https://pubmed.ncbi.nlm.nih.gov/21953338/.
https://pubmed.ncbi.nlm.nih.gov/26293764/.

344. Articles: https://pubmed.ncbi.nlm.nih.gov/26835300/.
https://pubmed.ncbi.nlm.nih.gov/36945996/. https://pubmed.ncbi.nlm.nih.gov/27251108/.
https://pubmed.ncbi.nlm.nih.gov/27375053/. https://pubmed.ncbi.nlm.nih.gov/29287191/.
https://pubmed.ncbi.nlm.nih.gov/33110622/. https://pubmed.ncbi.nlm.nih.gov/37432271/.

345. Related articles: https://pubmed.ncbi.nlm.nih.gov/36625789/.
https://pubmed.ncbi.nlm.nih.gov/29719821/. https://pubmed.ncbi.nlm.nih.gov/27876139/.

346. Articles: https://pubmed.ncbi.nlm.nih.gov/27088925/.
https://pubmed.ncbi.nlm.nih.gov/35218301/. https://pubmed.ncbi.nlm.nih.gov/26721572/.
https://pubmed.ncbi.nlm.nih.gov/39037099/. https://pubmed.ncbi.nlm.nih.gov/34396419/.
https://pubmed.ncbi.nlm.nih.gov/36192561/. https://pubmed.ncbi.nlm.nih.gov/24864027/.

347. Articles: https://pubmed.ncbi.nlm.nih.gov/38622859/.
https://pubmed.ncbi.nlm.nih.gov/25785742/. https://pubmed.ncbi.nlm.nih.gov/33307795/.
https://pubmed.ncbi.nlm.nih.gov/30843446/. https://pubmed.ncbi.nlm.nih.gov/24667068/.

348. Articles: https://pubmed.ncbi.nlm.nih.gov/32172354/.
https://pubmed.ncbi.nlm.nih.gov/21419275/. https://pubmed.ncbi.nlm.nih.gov/29846166/.
https://pubmed.ncbi.nlm.nih.gov/27179106/.

349. Article: https://pubmed.ncbi.nlm.nih.gov/31011257/.

350. Articles: https://www.ncbi.nlm.nih.gov/pmc/articles/PMC7584818/.
https://www.ncbi.nlm.nih.gov/pmc/articles/PMC5143473/.

351. Article: https://pubmed.ncbi.nlm.nih.gov/35383823/. See also *Bottom Line's 2021 Health Breakthroughs*, p. 304.

352. Articles: https://pubmed.ncbi.nlm.nih.gov/33590380/.
https://pubmed.ncbi.nlm.nih.gov/38348080/. https://pubmed.ncbi.nlm.nih.gov/37943388/.
https://pubmed.ncbi.nlm.nih.gov/27499590/. https://pubmed.ncbi.nlm.nih.gov/31905893/.
https://pubmed.ncbi.nlm.nih.gov/35546270/. https://pubmed.ncbi.nlm.nih.gov/30858945/.

353. Articles: https://pubmed.ncbi.nlm.nih.gov/37454668/.
https://pubmed.ncbi.nlm.nih.gov/34717822/.

354. Articles: https://pubmed.ncbi.nlm.nih.gov/36771474/.
https://pubmed.ncbi.nlm.nih.gov/35160157/. https://pubmed.ncbi.nlm.nih.gov/35440329/.
https://pubmed.ncbi.nlm.nih.gov/29022676/. https://pubmed.ncbi.nlm.nih.gov/34408425/.

355. Articles: https://pubmed.ncbi.nlm.nih.gov/36366796/.
https://www.nature.com/articles/s41598-021-99952-z.
https://pubmed.ncbi.nlm.nih.gov/32679589/. Studies show that those deficient in vitamin D are at
greater risk for infection. *Bottom Line's 2021 Health Breakthroughs*, p. 249.
356. Articles: https://pubmed.ncbi.nlm.nih.gov/24246682/.
https://pubmed.ncbi.nlm.nih.gov/34913244/.
357. Article: https://pubmed.ncbi.nlm.nih.gov/22761623/.
358. Articles: https://pubmed.ncbi.nlm.nih.gov/35198149/.
https://pubmed.ncbi.nlm.nih.gov/36607880/. https://pubmed.ncbi.nlm.nih.gov/26821547/.
https://pubmed.ncbi.nlm.nih.gov/33308613/.
359. Articles: https://pubmed.ncbi.nlm.nih.gov/36366796/.
https://pubmed.ncbi.nlm.nih.gov/32679589/. Studies show that those deficient in vitamin D are at
greater risk for infection. *Bottom Line's 2021 Health Breakthroughs*, p. 249.
360. Related articles: https://www.ncbi.nlm.nih.gov/pmc/articles/PMC7983154/.
https://aacrjournals.org/cancerpreventionresearch/article/3/10/1246/48846/Dietary-Vitamin-D-Exp
osure-Prevents-Obesity.
361. Articles:
https://pubmed.ncbi.nlm.nih.gov/31518608/#:~:text=population%2Dbased%20sample-,Posttrauma
tic%20stress%20disorder%20is%20associated%20with%20reduced%20vitamin%20D%20levels,Jan%20
10%3A96%3A109760.
https://www.psychiatrictimes.com/view/exploring-integrative-medicine-and-nutrition-for-ptsd.
https://foodforthebrain.org/ptsd/.
362. Articles: https://pubmed.ncbi.nlm.nih.gov/34421819/.
https://pubmed.ncbi.nlm.nih.gov/6265607/. https://pubmed.ncbi.nlm.nih.gov/13591293/.
https://pubmed.ncbi.nlm.nih.gov/38048414/.
363. Article: https://pubmed.ncbi.nlm.nih.gov/33396382/.
364. Articles: https://pubmed.ncbi.nlm.nih.gov/36184023/.
https://pubmed.ncbi.nlm.nih.gov/36894281/. https://pubmed.ncbi.nlm.nih.gov/27060679/.
https://pubmed.ncbi.nlm.nih.gov/24244212/.
365. Articles: https://pubmed.ncbi.nlm.nih.gov/32631584/.
https://pubmed.ncbi.nlm.nih.gov/35757436/. https://pubmed.ncbi.nlm.nih.gov/37261184/.
https://pubmed.ncbi.nlm.nih.gov/37745145/. https://pubmed.ncbi.nlm.nih.gov/6977549/.
https://pubmed.ncbi.nlm.nih.gov/19095601/.
366. Related articles: https://pubmed.ncbi.nlm.nih.gov/28807865/.
https://www.ncbi.nlm.nih.gov/books/NBK343782/. https://pubmed.ncbi.nlm.nih.gov/41816/.
367. Article: https://pubmed.ncbi.nlm.nih.gov/30415629/. See also Ryan, pp. 81-85.
368. Article: https://pubmed.ncbi.nlm.nih.gov/31679731/.
369. Articles: https://pubmed.ncbi.nlm.nih.gov/34290783/.
https://pubmed.ncbi.nlm.nih.gov/32490740/. https://pubmed.ncbi.nlm.nih.gov/31671292/.
https://pubmed.ncbi.nlm.nih.gov/34355550/. https://pubmed.ncbi.nlm.nih.gov/16469037/.
370. Articles: https://pubmed.ncbi.nlm.nih.gov/33217765/.
https://pubmed.ncbi.nlm.nih.gov/35458211/.
371. Articles: https://www.ncbi.nlm.nih.gov/pmc/articles/PMC10352003/.
https://www.healthline.com/nutrition/vitamin-deficiency.
372. Articles: https://pubmed.ncbi.nlm.nih.gov/6788286/.
https://pubmed.ncbi.nlm.nih.gov/6602194/. https://pubmed.ncbi.nlm.nih.gov/3976850/.
https://pubmed.ncbi.nlm.nih.gov/6620490/. https://pubmed.ncbi.nlm.nih.gov/26156834/.
373. Articles: https://pubmed.ncbi.nlm.nih.gov/34926545/.
https://pubmed.ncbi.nlm.nih.gov/24971035/. https://pubmed.ncbi.nlm.nih.gov/27177705/.
https://pubmed.ncbi.nlm.nih.gov/33485122/. https://pubmed.ncbi.nlm.nih.gov/34076230/.
https://pubmed.ncbi.nlm.nih.gov/34202164/. https://pubmed.ncbi.nlm.nih.gov/32938758/.
374. Articles: https://pubmed.ncbi.nlm.nih.gov/37457393/.
https://pubmed.ncbi.nlm.nih.gov/20144597/. https://pubmed.ncbi.nlm.nih.gov/28734792/.
https://pubmed.ncbi.nlm.nih.gov/36864582/.
375. Articles: https://pubmed.ncbi.nlm.nih.gov/32149392/.
https://pubmed.ncbi.nlm.nih.gov/27827293/. https://pubmed.ncbi.nlm.nih.gov/33987118/.
376. Related article: https://pubmed.ncbi.nlm.nih.gov/32672533/.

377. Articles: https://pubmed.ncbi.nlm.nih.gov/32359712/.
https://pubmed.ncbi.nlm.nih.gov/36753475/. https://pubmed.ncbi.nlm.nih.gov/38214845/.
https://pubmed.ncbi.nlm.nih.gov/30770428/. https://pubmed.ncbi.nlm.nih.gov/35255352/.
https://pubmed.ncbi.nlm.nih.gov/33071932/. https://pubmed.ncbi.nlm.nih.gov/35868492/.
378. Related articles: https://pubmed.ncbi.nlm.nih.gov/3516863/.
https://pubmed.ncbi.nlm.nih.gov/6182580/. https://pubmed.ncbi.nlm.nih.gov/16526182/.
https://pubmed.ncbi.nlm.nih.gov/7394200/.
379. Articles: https://pubmed.ncbi.nlm.nih.gov/33049684/.
https://pubmed.ncbi.nlm.nih.gov/35268010/. https://pubmed.ncbi.nlm.nih.gov/27116242/.
380. Articles: https://pubmed.ncbi.nlm.nih.gov/1652746/.
https://pubmed.ncbi.nlm.nih.gov/22319799/. https://pubmed.ncbi.nlm.nih.gov/35533340/.
https://pubmed.ncbi.nlm.nih.gov/29947083/. https://pubmed.ncbi.nlm.nih.gov/30711691/.
381. Related articles: https://pubmed.ncbi.nlm.nih.gov/?term=vitamin+d++dental+agenesis.
https://www.sciencedirect.com/science/article/pii/S2475299122130027#:~:text=Conclusion,stages
%20of%20the%20mandibular%20teeth. https://pubmed.ncbi.nlm.nih.gov/19021896/.
382. Articles: https://pubmed.ncbi.nlm.nih.gov/30344276/.
https://pubmed.ncbi.nlm.nih.gov/26860322/. https://pubmed.ncbi.nlm.nih.gov/30648367/.
Vitamin D is linked to bone and tooth development and strengthening. Weiss, p. 117.
383. Related article: https://pubmed.ncbi.nlm.nih.gov/11773605/.
384. Articles: https://pubmed.ncbi.nlm.nih.gov/31826364/.
https://pubmed.ncbi.nlm.nih.gov/36509315/.
https://www.ncbi.nlm.nih.gov/pmc/articles/PMC4511535/. A number of studies have linked
depression with vitamin D deficiency. Altshul and Hops, p. 225.
385. Article: https://pubmed.ncbi.nlm.nih.gov/27918470/.
386. Articles: https://pubmed.ncbi.nlm.nih.gov/25905277/.
https://pubmed.ncbi.nlm.nih.gov/27760369/. https://pubmed.ncbi.nlm.nih.gov/1846069/.
https://pubmed.ncbi.nlm.nih.gov/13584272/.
387. Article:
https://www.webmd.com/vitamins-and-supplements/what-to-know-about-vitamin-d-and-mental-healt
h.
388. Article: https://pubmed.ncbi.nlm.nih.gov/9094891/.
389. Articles: https://pubmed.ncbi.nlm.nih.gov/33413534/.
https://pubmed.ncbi.nlm.nih.gov/30262704/. https://pubmed.ncbi.nlm.nih.gov/17598904/.
390. Articles: https://pubmed.ncbi.nlm.nih.gov/24582099/.
https://pubmed.ncbi.nlm.nih.gov/36790836/. https://pubmed.ncbi.nlm.nih.gov/36835159/.
Vitamin D decreases inflammation and improves insulin resistance. Thus one Indian study found that
those who took vitamin D supplements were far less likely to develop prediabetes. God-Given Remedies, p.
110. See also Dowd and Stafford, pp. 130-131; Somerville, pp. 121-124.
391. Article:
https://omegaquant.com/can-low-vitamin-d-cause-neuropathy/#:~:text=BLOG%3A%20How%20to
%20Choose%20the,the%20hands%20and%2For%20feet.
392. Articles: https://pubmed.ncbi.nlm.nih.gov/37569392/.
https://pubmed.ncbi.nlm.nih.gov/35457041/. https://pubmed.ncbi.nlm.nih.gov/33026598/.
https://pubmed.ncbi.nlm.nih.gov/37085359/. https://pubmed.ncbi.nlm.nih.gov/33760363/.
https://pubmed.ncbi.nlm.nih.gov/28457295/.
https://eyesoneyecare.com/resources/ocular-manifestations-vitamin-deficiencies/.
393. Article: https://pubmed.ncbi.nlm.nih.gov/36918811/.
394. Articles: https://pubmed.ncbi.nlm.nih.gov/26496000/.
https://pubmed.ncbi.nlm.nih.gov/16121806/.
395. Article: https://pubmed.ncbi.nlm.nih.gov/27915988/.
396. Articles: https://pubmed.ncbi.nlm.nih.gov/35338644/.
https://pubmed.ncbi.nlm.nih.gov/33987118/. https://pubmed.ncbi.nlm.nih.gov/32045288/.
397. Related articles: https://pubmed.ncbi.nlm.nih.gov/35682491/.
https://pubmed.ncbi.nlm.nih.gov/32384728/.
398. Articles: https://pubmed.ncbi.nlm.nih.gov/30480416/.
https://pubmed.ncbi.nlm.nih.gov/10462240/. https://pubmed.ncbi.nlm.nih.gov/22854622/.
https://pubmed.ncbi.nlm.nih.gov/26678919/.

399. Articles: https://pubmed.ncbi.nlm.nih.gov/37868452/.
https://pubmed.ncbi.nlm.nih.gov/30356314/. https://pubmed.ncbi.nlm.nih.gov/31127184/.
https://pubmed.ncbi.nlm.nih.gov/12429765/. https://pubmed.ncbi.nlm.nih.gov/34323449/.
400. Article: https://pubmed.ncbi.nlm.nih.gov/25117159/.
401. Articles: https://pubmed.ncbi.nlm.nih.gov/31393320/.
https://www.ohsu.edu/sites/default/files/2019-08/Vitamin-mineral%20treatment%20improves%20a
ggression%20and%20emotional%20regulation%20in%20children%20with%20ADHD.pdf.
402. Articles: https://pubmed.ncbi.nlm.nih.gov/33551489/.
https://pubmed.ncbi.nlm.nih.gov/33604809/. https://pubmed.ncbi.nlm.nih.gov/34744508/.
403. Articles: https://pubmed.ncbi.nlm.nih.gov/38589451/.
https://www.nature.com/articles/s41598-024-58083-x.
https://www.researchgate.net/publication/379667618_Bone_mineral_density_in_adults_with_arthro
gryposis_multiplex_congenita_a_retrospective_cohort_analysis.
404. Articles: https://pubmed.ncbi.nlm.nih.gov/35934687/.
https://pubmed.ncbi.nlm.nih.gov/32919816/. https://pubmed.ncbi.nlm.nih.gov/25979437/.
https://pubmed.ncbi.nlm.nih.gov/27981318/.https://pubmed.ncbi.nlm.nih.gov/36795135/.
405. Articles: https://pubmed.ncbi.nlm.nih.gov/?term=vitamin+d+Diverticulitis.
https://pubmed.ncbi.nlm.nih.gov/23954650/. https://pubmed.ncbi.nlm.nih.gov/26251177/.
https://pubmed.ncbi.nlm.nih.gov/34690298/.
406. Articles: https://pubmed.ncbi.nlm.nih.gov/32759193/.
https://pubmed.ncbi.nlm.nih.gov/33231724/. https://pubmed.ncbi.nlm.nih.gov/37807761/.
407. Articles: https://pubmed.ncbi.nlm.nih.gov/31784293/.
https://pubmed.ncbi.nlm.nih.gov/37880588/. https://pubmed.ncbi.nlm.nih.gov/28571965/.
https://pubmed.ncbi.nlm.nih.gov/1535819/. https://pubmed.ncbi.nlm.nih.gov/34917171/.
https://pubmed.ncbi.nlm.nih.gov/25685147/.
408. Article:
https://omegaquant.com/can-low-vitamin-d-cause-neuropathy/#:~:text=BLOG%3A%20How%20to
%20Choose%20the,the%20hands%20and%2For%20feet.
409. Some people taking high dosages of vitamin D3 (along with magnesium and vitamin K2) report an
improvement in dream quality, describing them as more "pleasant" than usual. I have experienced the
same thing. L.S. See Bowles, pp. 89-90. Conversely, more nightmares are reported in individuals with a
deficiency of vitamin D. See article: https://pubmed.ncbi.nlm.nih.gov/34568104/.
410. Articles: https://pubmed.ncbi.nlm.nih.gov/36674972/.
https://pubmed.ncbi.nlm.nih.gov/32461421/. https://pubmed.ncbi.nlm.nih.gov/26269110/.
https://pubmed.ncbi.nlm.nih.gov/37026244/.
411. Articles: https://pubmed.ncbi.nlm.nih.gov/25905277/.
https://pubmed.ncbi.nlm.nih.gov/27760369/. https://pubmed.ncbi.nlm.nih.gov/1846069/.
https://pubmed.ncbi.nlm.nih.gov/13584272/.
412. Related articles: https://pubmed.ncbi.nlm.nih.gov/33407964/.
https://pubmed.ncbi.nlm.nih.gov/21060025/.
413. Article: https://pubmed.ncbi.nlm.nih.gov/27651381/.
414. Articles: https://pubmed.ncbi.nlm.nih.gov/37811112/.
https://pubmed.ncbi.nlm.nih.gov/37691106/. https://pubmed.ncbi.nlm.nih.gov/38877334/.
415. Articles: https://pubmed.ncbi.nlm.nih.gov/31940621/.
https://pubmed.ncbi.nlm.nih.gov/35334962/. https://pubmed.ncbi.nlm.nih.gov/30982641/.
https://pubmed.ncbi.nlm.nih.gov/34181909/.
416. Articles: https://pubmed.ncbi.nlm.nih.gov/32365423/.
https://pubmed.ncbi.nlm.nih.gov/23568194/. https://pubmed.ncbi.nlm.nih.gov/32193537/.
https://pubmed.ncbi.nlm.nih.gov/26027439/.
417. Articles: https://pubmed.ncbi.nlm.nih.gov/27809427/.
https://pubmed.ncbi.nlm.nih.gov/30370040/.https://pubmed.ncbi.nlm.nih.gov/24592758/.
418. Articles: https://pubmed.ncbi.nlm.nih.gov/23340562/.
https://pubmed.ncbi.nlm.nih.gov/30056817/. https://pubmed.ncbi.nlm.nih.gov/18806552/.
419. Article:
https://www.webmd.com/vitamins-and-supplements/what-to-know-about-vitamin-d-and-mental-healt
h.
420. Articles: https://pubmed.ncbi.nlm.nih.gov/25130505/.
https://pubmed.ncbi.nlm.nih.gov/10475815/.

421. Articles: https://www.ncbi.nlm.nih.gov/pmc/articles/PMC7058859/.
https://pubmed.ncbi.nlm.nih.gov/26029837/. https://pubmed.ncbi.nlm.nih.gov/33733568/.
422. Articles: https://pubmed.ncbi.nlm.nih.gov/36994022/.
https://pubmed.ncbi.nlm.nih.gov/32201492/. https://pubmed.ncbi.nlm.nih.gov/32851663/.
https://pubmed.ncbi.nlm.nih.gov/33173424/. https://pubmed.ncbi.nlm.nih.gov/37223025/.
423. Article: https://pubmed.ncbi.nlm.nih.gov/26239464/.
424. Articles: https://pubmed.ncbi.nlm.nih.gov/27488172/.
https://pubmed.ncbi.nlm.nih.gov/29511428/. https://pubmed.ncbi.nlm.nih.gov/27084695/.
https://pubmed.ncbi.nlm.nih.gov/30554346/.
425. Articles: https://pubmed.ncbi.nlm.nih.gov/26752631/.
https://journals.plos.org/plosone/article?id=10.1371/journal.pone.0145908.
426. Articles: https://pubmed.ncbi.nlm.nih.gov/27488172/.
https://pubmed.ncbi.nlm.nih.gov/29511428/. https://pubmed.ncbi.nlm.nih.gov/27084695/.
https://pubmed.ncbi.nlm.nih.gov/30554346/.
427. Article: https://pubmed.ncbi.nlm.nih.gov/29042303/.
428. Article: https://pubmed.ncbi.nlm.nih.gov/32056836/.
429. Related articles: https://pubmed.ncbi.nlm.nih.gov/32200644/.
https://pubmed.ncbi.nlm.nih.gov/35535019/.
430. Articles: https://pubmed.ncbi.nlm.nih.gov/?term=VITAMIN+d+Endometrial+Cancer.
https://pubmed.ncbi.nlm.nih.gov/18155758/. https://pubmed.ncbi.nlm.nih.gov/23136228/.
https://pubmed.ncbi.nlm.nih.gov/32483402/. https://pubmed.ncbi.nlm.nih.gov/17475316/.
https://pubmed.ncbi.nlm.nih.gov/29113037/.
431. Articles: https://pubmed.ncbi.nlm.nih.gov/37644533/.
https://pubmed.ncbi.nlm.nih.gov/36578019/. https://pubmed.ncbi.nlm.nih.gov/32453393/.
https://pubmed.ncbi.nlm.nih.gov/38698459/.
432. Articles: https://pubmed.ncbi.nlm.nih.gov/37447353/.
https://pubmed.ncbi.nlm.nih.gov/36246136/. https://pubmed.ncbi.nlm.nih.gov/32272973/.
433. Articles:
https://www.ncl.ac.uk/press/articles/archive/2013/04/vitamindproventoboostenergyfromwithinthec
ells.html. https://www.ncbi.nlm.nih.gov/pmc/articles/PMC4158648/.
https://www.livescience.com/does-vitamin-d-give-you-energy.
434. Related article: https://pubmed.ncbi.nlm.nih.gov/17200157/.
435. Articles: https://pubmed.ncbi.nlm.nih.gov/29598883/.
https://pubmed.ncbi.nlm.nih.gov/38857176/. https://pubmed.ncbi.nlm.nih.gov/30392888/.
https://pubmed.ncbi.nlm.nih.gov/24911026/.
436. Articles: https://pubmed.ncbi.nlm.nih.gov/37015752/.
https://pubmed.ncbi.nlm.nih.gov/19797953/. https://pubmed.ncbi.nlm.nih.gov/38183560/.
https://pubmed.ncbi.nlm.nih.gov/26004426/.
437. Articles: https://pubmed.ncbi.nlm.nih.gov/35961936/.
https://pubmed.ncbi.nlm.nih.gov/30074926/. https://pubmed.ncbi.nlm.nih.gov/37046594/.
https://pubmed.ncbi.nlm.nih.gov/37840401/. https://pubmed.ncbi.nlm.nih.gov/30133868/.
https://pubmed.ncbi.nlm.nih.gov/26365559/.
438. Articles: https://pubmed.ncbi.nlm.nih.gov/28947637/.
https://pubmed.ncbi.nlm.nih.gov/27988507/. https://pubmed.ncbi.nlm.nih.gov/24063762/.
https://pubmed.ncbi.nlm.nih.gov/29399794/. https://pubmed.ncbi.nlm.nih.gov/24738630/.
https://pubmed.ncbi.nlm.nih.gov/32363640/.
439. Articles: https://pubmed.ncbi.nlm.nih.gov/29537299/.
https://pubmed.ncbi.nlm.nih.gov/27619037/. https://pubmed.ncbi.nlm.nih.gov/28648890/.
https://pubmed.ncbi.nlm.nih.gov/28647162/. https://pubmed.ncbi.nlm.nih.gov/22311466/.
440. Articles: https://pubmed.ncbi.nlm.nih.gov/33834708/.
https://pubmed.ncbi.nlm.nih.gov/27505106/. https://pubmed.ncbi.nlm.nih.gov/26046559/.
https://pubmed.ncbi.nlm.nih.gov/21864064/.
441. Articles: https://pubmed.ncbi.nlm.nih.gov/37371510/.
https://pubmed.ncbi.nlm.nih.gov/25092061/. https://pubmed.ncbi.nlm.nih.gov/32725942/.
https://pubmed.ncbi.nlm.nih.gov/32009309/. https://pubmed.ncbi.nlm.nih.gov/30523636/.
442. Articles: https://www.ncbi.nlm.nih.gov/pmc/articles/PMC6493208/. Related article:
https://sunsaferx.com/blogs/health-wellness/erythema-treatment-prevention.

443. Articles: https://pubmed.ncbi.nlm.nih.gov/34763310/.
https://pubmed.ncbi.nlm.nih.gov/24137761/. https://pubmed.ncbi.nlm.nih.gov/23536284/.
https://pubmed.ncbi.nlm.nih.gov/38634774/. https://pubmed.ncbi.nlm.nih.gov/18476956/.
https://pubmed.ncbi.nlm.nih.gov/20412370/. https://www.ncbi.nlm.nih.gov/books/NBK563141/.
444. Article: https://pubmed.ncbi.nlm.nih.gov/25590952/.
445. Articles: https://pubmed.ncbi.nlm.nih.gov/6438480/.
https://pubmed.ncbi.nlm.nih.gov/31784293/.
446. Articles: https://pubmed.ncbi.nlm.nih.gov/35767173/.
https://pubmed.ncbi.nlm.nih.gov/31831865/. https://pubmed.ncbi.nlm.nih.gov/31177660/.
https://pubmed.ncbi.nlm.nih.gov/1944002/.
447. Articles: https://pubmed.ncbi.nlm.nih.gov/31082167/.
https://pubmed.ncbi.nlm.nih.gov/3521493/.
448. Articles: https://pubmed.ncbi.nlm.nih.gov/19669759/.
https://www.mdpi.com/2072-6643/15/21/4571. https://pubmed.ncbi.nlm.nih.gov/14528100/.
https://pubmed.ncbi.nlm.nih.gov/22806259/.
https://www.cancertherapyadvisor.com/news/vitamin-d-supplementation-recommended-for-pediatric
-patients-with-sarcoma/. https://www.ncbi.nlm.nih.gov/pmc/articles/PMC9313306/.
https://www.oncologynurseadvisor.com/news/vitamin-d-supplementation-is-recommended-for-use-in
-young-patients-with-sarcoma/.
449. Article:
https://www.kairoswellnesscollective.com/blog/best-supplements-for-skin-picking-disorder.
450. Articles: https://pubmed.ncbi.nlm.nih.gov/29351464/.
https://pubmed.ncbi.nlm.nih.gov/35684153/. https://pubmed.ncbi.nlm.nih.gov/32169320/.
https://pubmed.ncbi.nlm.nih.gov/31741672/. https://pubmed.ncbi.nlm.nih.gov/22632164/.
451. Article: https://pubmed.ncbi.nlm.nih.gov/30467438/.
452. Articles: https://pubmed.ncbi.nlm.nih.gov/35961936/.
https://pubmed.ncbi.nlm.nih.gov/30074926/. https://pubmed.ncbi.nlm.nih.gov/37046594/.
https://pubmed.ncbi.nlm.nih.gov/37840401/. https://pubmed.ncbi.nlm.nih.gov/30133868/.
https://pubmed.ncbi.nlm.nih.gov/26365559/.
453. Articles: https://pubmed.ncbi.nlm.nih.gov/29317405/.
https://pubmed.ncbi.nlm.nih.gov/32328382/.
454. Articles: https://pubmed.ncbi.nlm.nih.gov/30430526/.
https://pubmed.ncbi.nlm.nih.gov/37284033/. https://pubmed.ncbi.nlm.nih.gov/35864655/.
https://pubmed.ncbi.nlm.nih.gov/27184385/.
455. Article: https://pubmed.ncbi.nlm.nih.gov/27494391/. See also Zaidi, p. 181.
456. Articles: https://pubmed.ncbi.nlm.nih.gov/20043299/.
https://pubmed.ncbi.nlm.nih.gov/27768599/. https://pubmed.ncbi.nlm.nih.gov/30983515/.
https://pubmed.ncbi.nlm.nih.gov/36334333/. https://pubmed.ncbi.nlm.nih.gov/19035286/.
https://pubmed.ncbi.nlm.nih.gov/25597951/.
457. Article: https://pubmed.ncbi.nlm.nih.gov/24450309/.
458. Article: https://pubmed.ncbi.nlm.nih.gov/16121806/.
459. Articles: https://pubmed.ncbi.nlm.nih.gov/20301575/.
https://pubmed.ncbi.nlm.nih.gov/32397406/. https://pubmed.ncbi.nlm.nih.gov/13155609/.
https://pubmed.ncbi.nlm.nih.gov/13610080/.
460. Article: https://pubmed.ncbi.nlm.nih.gov/21258262/. See also Bowles, p. 62.
461. Article: https://pubmed.ncbi.nlm.nih.gov/38257114/. See also Khalsa, pp. 129-130.
462. Articles: https://www.ncbi.nlm.nih.gov/pmc/articles/PMC2839878/.
https://www.ncbi.nlm.nih.gov/pmc/articles/PMC8159757/.
https://onlinelibrary.wiley.com/doi/10.1155/2020/2656321.
463. Articles: https://pubmed.ncbi.nlm.nih.gov/36980086/.
https://pubmed.ncbi.nlm.nih.gov/32110543/. https://pubmed.ncbi.nlm.nih.gov/38143518/.
https://pubmed.ncbi.nlm.nih.gov/34336337/. https://pubmed.ncbi.nlm.nih.gov/15707811/.
464. See also bowel incontinence. Article: https://pubmed.ncbi.nlm.nih.gov/38316640/.
465. Article: https://pubmed.ncbi.nlm.nih.gov/34747902/.
466. Articles: https://pubmed.ncbi.nlm.nih.gov/24816220/.
https://pubmed.ncbi.nlm.nih.gov/33232716/. https://pubmed.ncbi.nlm.nih.gov/23104117/.
https://pubmed.ncbi.nlm.nih.gov/8176126/.

467. Articles: https://pubmed.ncbi.nlm.nih.gov/35198149/.
https://pubmed.ncbi.nlm.nih.gov/36388314/. https://pubmed.ncbi.nlm.nih.gov/36299453/.
https://pubmed.ncbi.nlm.nih.gov/32940108/.
468. Articles: https://pubmed.ncbi.nlm.nih.gov/33851285/.
https://pubmed.ncbi.nlm.nih.gov/30343406/. https://pubmed.ncbi.nlm.nih.gov/31041177/.
469. Articles: https://pubmed.ncbi.nlm.nih.gov/37266579/.
https://pubmed.ncbi.nlm.nih.gov/36344288/. https://pubmed.ncbi.nlm.nih.gov/35960442/.
https://pubmed.ncbi.nlm.nih.gov/30011902/. https://pubmed.ncbi.nlm.nih.gov/33743958/.
https://pubmed.ncbi.nlm.nih.gov/33108619/. https://pubmed.ncbi.nlm.nih.gov/32033736/.
470. Article: https://pubmed.ncbi.nlm.nih.gov/36591895/.
471. Article: https://pubmed.ncbi.nlm.nih.gov/34188748/.
472. Article: https://pubmed.ncbi.nlm.nih.gov/32252338/. Because vitamin D strengthens the
immune system by energizing natural antibodies, it can help fight off the common cold. *God-Given
Remedies*, p. 72.
473. Articles: https://pubmed.ncbi.nlm.nih.gov/35241255/.
https://www.ncbi.nlm.nih.gov/pmc/articles/PMC9820561/.
https://www.medlink.com/articles/vitamin-d-in-neurologic-disorders.
https://www.clinicaladvisor.com/features/vitamin-d-deficiency-neurologic-disorders/#:~:text=Altho
ugh%20decades%20of%20research%20suggest,management%20of%20these%20conditions%20is.
https://www.ncbi.nlm.nih.gov/pmc/articles/PMC6121649/.
474. Article:
https://www.webmd.com/vitamins-and-supplements/what-to-know-about-vitamin-d-and-mental-healt
h.
475. Articles: https://pubmed.ncbi.nlm.nih.gov/28039109/.
https://www.webmd.com/vitamins-and-supplements/what-to-know-about-vitamin-d-and-mental-healt
h.
476. Article: https://pubmed.ncbi.nlm.nih.gov/25558907/.
477. Articles: https://pubmed.ncbi.nlm.nih.gov/25829979/.
https://pubmed.ncbi.nlm.nih.gov/33924232/. https://pubmed.ncbi.nlm.nih.gov/28441981/.
478. Articles: https://pubmed.ncbi.nlm.nih.gov/32556549/.
https://pubmed.ncbi.nlm.nih.gov/22715859/.
479. Article: https://pubmed.ncbi.nlm.nih.gov/22715859/.
480. Articles: https://pubmed.ncbi.nlm.nih.gov/33045979/.
https://pubmed.ncbi.nlm.nih.gov/37194326/.
481. Articles: https://pubmed.ncbi.nlm.nih.gov/30017798/.
https://pubmed.ncbi.nlm.nih.gov/32741494/.
https://www.ncbi.nlm.nih.gov/pmc/articles/PMC8058406/.
482. In my personal experience the condition known as "frozen shoulder" may sometimes be caused by a
vitamin D deficiency. L.S. Articles: https://pubmed.ncbi.nlm.nih.gov/15182797/.
https://www.careatc.com/improving-health/the-link-between-shoulder-pain-and-vitamin-d-deficiency.
https://pubmed.ncbi.nlm.nih.gov/30321335/. https://pubmed.ncbi.nlm.nih.gov/6387576/.
https://pubmed.ncbi.nlm.nih.gov/33390486/. https://pubmed.ncbi.nlm.nih.gov/7014108/.
https://annalsmedres.org/index.php/aomr/article/view/448.
https://www.tampabay.com/news/health/Mayo-Clinic-Q-A-treating-frozen-shoulder-calcium-supple
ments-versus-exercise_165896098/.
https://www.businessinsider.com/guides/health/treatments/frozen-shoulder.
483. Articles: https://pubmed.ncbi.nlm.nih.gov/37811112/.
https://pubmed.ncbi.nlm.nih.gov/37691106/. https://pubmed.ncbi.nlm.nih.gov/30386607/.
https://pubmed.ncbi.nlm.nih.gov/38877334/.
484. Articles: https://pubmed.ncbi.nlm.nih.gov/27915988/.
https://pubmed.ncbi.nlm.nih.gov/34766885/. https://pubmed.ncbi.nlm.nih.gov/31011257/.
https://pubmed.ncbi.nlm.nih.gov/30511197/.
485. Articles: https://pubmed.ncbi.nlm.nih.gov/35241255/.
https://www.ncbi.nlm.nih.gov/pmc/articles/PMC9820561/.
https://www.medlink.com/articles/vitamin-d-in-neurologic-disorders.
https://www.clinicaladvisor.com/features/vitamin-d-deficiency-neurologic-disorders/#:~:text=Altho
ugh%20decades%20of%20research%20suggest,management%20of%20these%20conditions%20is.
https://www.ncbi.nlm.nih.gov/pmc/articles/PMC6121649/.
486. Articles: https://pubmed.ncbi.nlm.nih.gov/38375518/.
https://pubmed.ncbi.nlm.nih.gov/27017390/. https://pubmed.ncbi.nlm.nih.gov/28672783/.

487. Articles: https://pubmed.ncbi.nlm.nih.gov/38572190/.
https://fasafw.com/blog/how-to-prevent-and-treat-toenail-fungus/.
https://www.ncbi.nlm.nih.gov/pmc/articles/PMC5537771/.
488. Articles: https://pubmed.ncbi.nlm.nih.gov/32117550/.
https://pubmed.ncbi.nlm.nih.gov/5613936/. https://pubmed.ncbi.nlm.nih.gov/3503543/.
https://pubmed.ncbi.nlm.nih.gov/37664264/.
489. Articles: https://pubmed.ncbi.nlm.nih.gov/20301691/.
https://pubmed.ncbi.nlm.nih.gov/10763902/. https://pubmed.ncbi.nlm.nih.gov/15454106/.
https://pubmed.ncbi.nlm.nih.gov/21779791/. https://pubmed.ncbi.nlm.nih.gov/27995581/.
https://pubmed.ncbi.nlm.nih.gov/16782422/.
490. Articles: https://pubmed.ncbi.nlm.nih.gov/32918214/.
https://pubmed.ncbi.nlm.nih.gov/31591986/. https://pubmed.ncbi.nlm.nih.gov/25078595/.
https://pubmed.ncbi.nlm.nih.gov/17540555/.
491. Articles: https://pubmed.ncbi.nlm.nih.gov/35068796/.
https://pubmed.ncbi.nlm.nih.gov/20301446/. https://pubmed.ncbi.nlm.nih.gov/26507741/.
https://pubmed.ncbi.nlm.nih.gov/27696253/. https://pubmed.ncbi.nlm.nih.gov/25078595/.
492. Bowles. pp. 72, 197, 198. See also articles: https://pubmed.ncbi.nlm.nih.gov/37002879/.
https://aventusclinic.com/the-relationship-between-ganglion-cysts-and-vitamin-d-deficiency/.
493. Article: https://pubmed.ncbi.nlm.nih.gov/2133956/.
494. Articles: https://pubmed.ncbi.nlm.nih.gov/30409113/.
https://pubmed.ncbi.nlm.nih.gov/21286859/. https://pubmed.ncbi.nlm.nih.gov/34881266/.
495. Articles: https://pubmed.ncbi.nlm.nih.gov/28906318/.
https://pubmed.ncbi.nlm.nih.gov/36566365/. https://pubmed.ncbi.nlm.nih.gov/31784293/.
496. Articles: https://pubmed.ncbi.nlm.nih.gov/25047396/.
https://pubmed.ncbi.nlm.nih.gov/33396382/. https://pubmed.ncbi.nlm.nih.gov/36868465/.
https://pubmed.ncbi.nlm.nih.gov/35100245/. https://pubmed.ncbi.nlm.nih.gov/29762159/.
497. Article:
https://med.virginia.edu/ginutrition/wp-content/uploads/sites/199/2015/11/JavorskyArticle-March
-06.pdf.
498. Articles: https://pubmed.ncbi.nlm.nih.gov/30972274/.
https://pubmed.ncbi.nlm.nih.gov/29981368/. https://pubmed.ncbi.nlm.nih.gov/36708580/.
https://pubmed.ncbi.nlm.nih.gov/27768599/. https://pubmed.ncbi.nlm.nih.gov/24013983/.
499. Article: https://pubmed.ncbi.nlm.nih.gov/32606868/.
500. Articles: https://pubmed.ncbi.nlm.nih.gov/20301446/.
https://pubmed.ncbi.nlm.nih.gov/31233632/. https://pubmed.ncbi.nlm.nih.gov/20920864/.
https://pubmed.ncbi.nlm.nih.gov/19147383/.
501. Articles: https://pubmed.ncbi.nlm.nih.gov/11096695/.
https://pubmed.ncbi.nlm.nih.gov/28138903/. https://pubmed.ncbi.nlm.nih.gov/14664769/.
https://pubmed.ncbi.nlm.nih.gov/33577006/. https://pubmed.ncbi.nlm.nih.gov/38169875/.
502. Related articles: https://pubmed.ncbi.nlm.nih.gov/34497118/.
https://pubmed.ncbi.nlm.nih.gov/36048500/. https://pubmed.ncbi.nlm.nih.gov/31405768/.
https://pubmed.ncbi.nlm.nih.gov/25739677/. https://pubmed.ncbi.nlm.nih.gov/32691168/.
https://pubmed.ncbi.nlm.nih.gov/28370342/.
503. Articles: https://pubmed.ncbi.nlm.nih.gov/31478182/.
https://pubmed.ncbi.nlm.nih.gov/35311615/. https://pubmed.ncbi.nlm.nih.gov/35156551/.
https://pubmed.ncbi.nlm.nih.gov/36558485/. https://pubmed.ncbi.nlm.nih.gov/36295786/.
504. Article: https://pubmed.ncbi.nlm.nih.gov/36901976/.
505. Articles: https://pubmed.ncbi.nlm.nih.gov/33550671/.
https://pubmed.ncbi.nlm.nih.gov/27730031/. https://pubmed.ncbi.nlm.nih.gov/33764502/.
506. Related articles: https://pubmed.ncbi.nlm.nih.gov/24933120/.
https://pubmed.ncbi.nlm.nih.gov/33113105/. https://pubmed.ncbi.nlm.nih.gov/26747961/.
507. Articles: https://pubmed.ncbi.nlm.nih.gov/28906318/.
https://pubmed.ncbi.nlm.nih.gov/36566365/. https://pubmed.ncbi.nlm.nih.gov/31784293/.
508. Articles: https://pubmed.ncbi.nlm.nih.gov/37114140/.
https://pubmed.ncbi.nlm.nih.gov/22213325/. https://pubmed.ncbi.nlm.nih.gov/23098692/.
509. Articles: https://pubmed.ncbi.nlm.nih.gov/36191611/.
https://pubmed.ncbi.nlm.nih.gov/31731439/. https://pubmed.ncbi.nlm.nih.gov/24277676/.
510. Related articles: https://pubmed.ncbi.nlm.nih.gov/38047239/.
https://pubmed.ncbi.nlm.nih.gov/35916795/. https://pubmed.ncbi.nlm.nih.gov/19688952/.

511. Articles: https://pubmed.ncbi.nlm.nih.gov/30017798/.
https://pubmed.ncbi.nlm.nih.gov/32741494/.
https://www.ncbi.nlm.nih.gov/pmc/articles/PMC8058406/.
512. Articles: https://pubmed.ncbi.nlm.nih.gov/35057450/.
https://pubmed.ncbi.nlm.nih.gov/36813995/.
513. Articles: https://pubmed.ncbi.nlm.nih.gov/11096695/.
https://pubmed.ncbi.nlm.nih.gov/28138903/. https://pubmed.ncbi.nlm.nih.gov/14664769/.
https://pubmed.ncbi.nlm.nih.gov/33577006/. https://pubmed.ncbi.nlm.nih.gov/38169875/.
514. Articles: https://pubmed.ncbi.nlm.nih.gov/37417841/.
https://pubmed.ncbi.nlm.nih.gov/2768861/.
515. Articles: https://pubmed.ncbi.nlm.nih.gov/31914014/.
https://pubmed.ncbi.nlm.nih.gov/39007836/. https://pubmed.ncbi.nlm.nih.gov/37694098/.
https://pubmed.ncbi.nlm.nih.gov/38124730/. https://pubmed.ncbi.nlm.nih.gov/32902920/.
https://pubmed.ncbi.nlm.nih.gov/32438644/.
516. Article: https://pubmed.ncbi.nlm.nih.gov/27505106/.
517. Article: https://www.ijpediatrics.com/index.php/ijcp/article/view/5488/3362.
518. Articles: https://pubmed.ncbi.nlm.nih.gov/35457041/.
https://pubmed.ncbi.nlm.nih.gov/33004198/. https://pubmed.ncbi.nlm.nih.gov/27980361/.
519. Articles: https://pubmed.ncbi.nlm.nih.gov/32117550/.
https://pubmed.ncbi.nlm.nih.gov/5613936/. https://pubmed.ncbi.nlm.nih.gov/3503543/.
https://pubmed.ncbi.nlm.nih.gov/37664264/.
520. Articles: https://pubmed.ncbi.nlm.nih.gov/20301788/.
https://pubmed.ncbi.nlm.nih.gov/20060350/. https://pubmed.ncbi.nlm.nih.gov/20060350/.
https://pubmed.ncbi.nlm.nih.gov/29960865/. https://pubmed.ncbi.nlm.nih.gov/34578865/.
521. Articles: https://pubmed.ncbi.nlm.nih.gov/35852202/.
https://pubmed.ncbi.nlm.nih.gov/38795863/.
522. Article: https://pubmed.ncbi.nlm.nih.gov/23642399/.
523. Article: https://pubmed.ncbi.nlm.nih.gov/32606868/.
524. Articles: https://pubmed.ncbi.nlm.nih.gov/24803734/.
https://pubmed.ncbi.nlm.nih.gov/24202285/.
525. Articles: https://pubmed.ncbi.nlm.nih.gov/34639000/.
https://pubmed.ncbi.nlm.nih.gov/30679908/.
526. Articles: https://pubmed.ncbi.nlm.nih.gov/32107168/.
https://pubmed.ncbi.nlm.nih.gov/32107168/. https://pubmed.ncbi.nlm.nih.gov/34064075/.
https://pubmed.ncbi.nlm.nih.gov/37218433/. https://pubmed.ncbi.nlm.nih.gov/26007334/.
https://pubmed.ncbi.nlm.nih.gov/36166168/. https://pubmed.ncbi.nlm.nih.gov/37505062/.
527. Articles: https://www.ncbi.nlm.nih.gov/pmc/articles/PMC7868724/.
528. Articles: https://pubmed.ncbi.nlm.nih.gov/31724740/.
https://pubmed.ncbi.nlm.nih.gov/31542066/. https://pubmed.ncbi.nlm.nih.gov/9649669/.
https://pubmed.ncbi.nlm.nih.gov/15506319/.
529. Articles: https://pubmed.ncbi.nlm.nih.gov/21575536/.
https://pubmed.ncbi.nlm.nih.gov/27417476/.
530. Article: https://pubmed.ncbi.nlm.nih.gov/30744880/.
531. Articles: https://pubmed.ncbi.nlm.nih.gov/35514132/.
https://pubmed.ncbi.nlm.nih.gov/35524469/. https://pubmed.ncbi.nlm.nih.gov/37557090/.
532. Articles: https://pubmed.ncbi.nlm.nih.gov/32438644/.
https://pubmed.ncbi.nlm.nih.gov/37312090/. https://pubmed.ncbi.nlm.nih.gov/31199730/.
533. Articles: https://pubmed.ncbi.nlm.nih.gov/37764988/.
https://pubmed.ncbi.nlm.nih.gov/29858878/.
534. Articles: https://pubmed.ncbi.nlm.nih.gov/36048921/.
https://pubmed.ncbi.nlm.nih.gov/25762358/. https://pubmed.ncbi.nlm.nih.gov/35941635/.
535. Related articles: https://pubmed.ncbi.nlm.nih.gov/32200644/.
https://pubmed.ncbi.nlm.nih.gov/35535019/.
536. Article: https://pubmed.ncbi.nlm.nih.gov/37908643/.
537. Articles: https://pubmed.ncbi.nlm.nih.gov/32252338/.
https://pubmed.ncbi.nlm.nih.gov/34827621/. https://pubmed.ncbi.nlm.nih.gov/22797987/.
https://pubmed.ncbi.nlm.nih.gov/37407993/.

538. Articles: https://pubmed.ncbi.nlm.nih.gov/25748421/.
https://pubmed.ncbi.nlm.nih.gov/22008469/.
539. Articles: https://pubmed.ncbi.nlm.nih.gov/34553483/.
https://pubmed.ncbi.nlm.nih.gov/30547302/. https://pubmed.ncbi.nlm.nih.gov/33642467/.
https://pubmed.ncbi.nlm.nih.gov/28508256/.
540. Related articles: https://pubmed.ncbi.nlm.nih.gov/26767392/.
https://pubmed.ncbi.nlm.nih.gov/25311777/. https://pubmed.ncbi.nlm.nih.gov/38292780/.
https://pubmed.ncbi.nlm.nih.gov/24803734/. https://pubmed.ncbi.nlm.nih.gov/23816059/.
541. Articles: https://pubmed.ncbi.nlm.nih.gov/30343406/.
https://www.anklefootmd.com/vitamin-d-can-boost-healing-following-bunion-surgery/.
https://www.bunionsurgeryspecialistsllc.com/vitamin-and-mineral-supplementation-for-bone-health/.
542. Articles: https://pubmed.ncbi.nlm.nih.gov/32556549/.
https://pubmed.ncbi.nlm.nih.gov/31587312/. https://pubmed.ncbi.nlm.nih.gov/30357860/.
https://pubmed.ncbi.nlm.nih.gov/28489032/. https://pubmed.ncbi.nlm.nih.gov/28943436/.
543. Articles: https://pubmed.ncbi.nlm.nih.gov/32899880/.
https://pubmed.ncbi.nlm.nih.gov/25144342/. https://pubmed.ncbi.nlm.nih.gov/28043680/.
544. Articles: https://pubmed.ncbi.nlm.nih.gov/28315909/.
https://pubmed.ncbi.nlm.nih.gov/37513592/. https://pubmed.ncbi.nlm.nih.gov/35563541/.
545. Articles: https://pubmed.ncbi.nlm.nih.gov/28487837/.
https://pubmed.ncbi.nlm.nih.gov/28102718/. https://pubmed.ncbi.nlm.nih.gov/27188226/.
https://pubmed.ncbi.nlm.nih.gov/34150589/. https://pubmed.ncbi.nlm.nih.gov/37716008/.
546. Articles: https://pubmed.ncbi.nlm.nih.gov/26156834/.
https://pubmed.ncbi.nlm.nih.gov/26800885/. https://pubmed.ncbi.nlm.nih.gov/35076925/.
https://pubmed.ncbi.nlm.nih.gov/31660939/.
547. Articles: https://pubmed.ncbi.nlm.nih.gov/29971976/.
https://pubmed.ncbi.nlm.nih.gov/37635492/. https://pubmed.ncbi.nlm.nih.gov/37738749/.
548. Articles: https://pubmed.ncbi.nlm.nih.gov/37299554/.
https://pubmed.ncbi.nlm.nih.gov/33216252/. https://pubmed.ncbi.nlm.nih.gov/33732250/.
https://pubmed.ncbi.nlm.nih.gov/32872541/. https://pubmed.ncbi.nlm.nih.gov/24564776/.
549. Articles: https://pubmed.ncbi.nlm.nih.gov/33247302/.
https://pubmed.ncbi.nlm.nih.gov/20301427/. https://pubmed.ncbi.nlm.nih.gov/31068690/. Lack of
vitamin D can cause the bones of the inner ear to become porous, inhibiting their ability to transmit
sound waves. *Smart Nutrition*, p. 41.
550. Articles: https://pubmed.ncbi.nlm.nih.gov/25705008/.
https://pubmed.ncbi.nlm.nih.gov/28384800/.
551. Article: https://pubmed.ncbi.nlm.nih.gov/34982819/. The heart needs calcium to function
correctly and vitamin D helps regulate the level of calcium in your blood. *Smart Nutrition*, p. 41.
552. Articles: https://pubmed.ncbi.nlm.nih.gov/23565451/.
https://pubmed.ncbi.nlm.nih.gov/29450171/. https://pubmed.ncbi.nlm.nih.gov/31496777/.
https://pubmed.ncbi.nlm.nih.gov/36694870/.
553. Articles: https://pubmed.ncbi.nlm.nih.gov/34684604/.
https://pubmed.ncbi.nlm.nih.gov/34464368/. https://pubmed.ncbi.nlm.nih.gov/18827580/.
554. Article: https://pubmed.ncbi.nlm.nih.gov/28808858/.
555. Articles: https://pubmed.ncbi.nlm.nih.gov/21631423/.
https://pubmed.ncbi.nlm.nih.gov/28817241/. https://pubmed.ncbi.nlm.nih.gov/30701749/.
556. Note that too little or too much vitamin D can cause heart palpitations in some individuals. L.S.
Articles: https://health.clevelandclinic.org/heart-palpitations-and-supplements.
https://omegaquant.com/how-does-vitamin-d-affect-your-heart/.
https://www.verywellhealth.com/taking-extra-vitamin-d-could-lower-risk-of-afib-7563876.
557. Articles: https://pubmed.ncbi.nlm.nih.gov/25485786/.
https://pubmed.ncbi.nlm.nih.gov/26825623/. https://pubmed.ncbi.nlm.nih.gov/32337015/.
558. Articles: https://pubmed.ncbi.nlm.nih.gov/30811162/.
https://www.ncbi.nlm.nih.gov/pmc/articles/PMC4192075/.
https://www.aafp.org/pubs/afp/issues/2019/0301/p285.html.
559. Articles: https://pubmed.ncbi.nlm.nih.gov/36411916/.
https://pubmed.ncbi.nlm.nih.gov/23396730/. https://pubmed.ncbi.nlm.nih.gov/29398866/.
https://pubmed.ncbi.nlm.nih.gov/36672644/. https://pubmed.ncbi.nlm.nih.gov/34295980/.
560. Articles: https://pubmed.ncbi.nlm.nih.gov/35126856/.
https://pubmed.ncbi.nlm.nih.gov/23016163/.

561. Articles: https://pubmed.ncbi.nlm.nih.gov/36411916/.
https://pubmed.ncbi.nlm.nih.gov/36672644/. https://pubmed.ncbi.nlm.nih.gov/29248582/.
https://pubmed.ncbi.nlm.nih.gov/31932201/.

562. Articles: https://pubmed.ncbi.nlm.nih.gov/29664746/.
https://pubmed.ncbi.nlm.nih.gov/34420582/. https://pubmed.ncbi.nlm.nih.gov/24124339/.
https://pubmed.ncbi.nlm.nih.gov/22189978/. https://pubmed.ncbi.nlm.nih.gov/26379820/.

563. Articles: https://pubmed.ncbi.nlm.nih.gov/37261280/.
https://pubmed.ncbi.nlm.nih.gov/25774877/. https://pubmed.ncbi.nlm.nih.gov/6815376/.
https://pubmed.ncbi.nlm.nih.gov/855812/.

564. Articles: https://pubmed.ncbi.nlm.nih.gov/31793406/.
https://pubmed.ncbi.nlm.nih.gov/33557624/. https://pubmed.ncbi.nlm.nih.gov/25299063/.
https://pubmed.ncbi.nlm.nih.gov/35957837/.

565. There is almost no doubt in my mind that a vitamin D deficiency contributes to the creation of reducible inguinal hernia due to the weakening of abdominal and inguinal muscles. *This is my theory*, and as I have written a book on inguinal hernia (see below), I have strong reason to believe this. I was later able to find only one medical study to support it: Article: https://www.researchgate.net/publication/340789860_Does_Vitamin_D_Deficiency_Cause_Direct_I nguinal_Hernia_Preliminary_Results. I also found a study that focuses on rats with diaphragmatic hernia (see below). Despite this, there are numerous scientific studies and reports linking vitamin D deficiency with weakening of the muscles, another reason I believe there is a connection. For example, see articles: https://pubmed.ncbi.nlm.nih.gov/29963601/. https://pubmed.ncbi.nlm.nih.gov/33484710/. https://pubmed.ncbi.nlm.nih.gov/11991436/. https://pubmed.ncbi.nlm.nih.gov/24867188/. https://pubmed.ncbi.nlm.nih.gov/31766576/. https://pubmed.ncbi.nlm.nih.gov/35595176/. For more information on self-treatment of reducible inguinal hernia, see my book *Victorian Hernia Cures*. L.S.

566. Articles: https://pubmed.ncbi.nlm.nih.gov/37868452/.
https://pubmed.ncbi.nlm.nih.gov/30356314/. https://pubmed.ncbi.nlm.nih.gov/31127184/.
https://pubmed.ncbi.nlm.nih.gov/12429765/. https://pubmed.ncbi.nlm.nih.gov/34323449/.

567. Article: https://pubmed.ncbi.nlm.nih.gov/31145049/.
https://pubmed.ncbi.nlm.nih.gov/37081493/.

568. Articles: https://pubmed.ncbi.nlm.nih.gov/36367186/.
https://pubmed.ncbi.nlm.nih.gov/29792782/. https://pubmed.ncbi.nlm.nih.gov/21269574/.
https://pubmed.ncbi.nlm.nih.gov/37081493/. https://pubmed.ncbi.nlm.nih.gov/31145049/.

569. Articles: https://pubmed.ncbi.nlm.nih.gov/33511224/.
https://pubmed.ncbi.nlm.nih.gov/35940884/. https://pubmed.ncbi.nlm.nih.gov/31594899/.

570. Articles: https://pubmed.ncbi.nlm.nih.gov/32899880/.
https://pubmed.ncbi.nlm.nih.gov/36902110/. https://pubmed.ncbi.nlm.nih.gov/31389312/. Low levels of vitamin D3 have been linked to hypertension. *Bottom Line's 2021 Health Breakthroughs*, p. 304.

571. Articles: https://pubmed.ncbi.nlm.nih.gov/33802330/.
https://pubmed.ncbi.nlm.nih.gov/36771474/. https://pubmed.ncbi.nlm.nih.gov/34954855/.
https://pubmed.ncbi.nlm.nih.gov/37779053/. https://pubmed.ncbi.nlm.nih.gov/29124703/.

572. Related article: https://pubmed.ncbi.nlm.nih.gov/11035908/.

573. Articles: https://pubmed.ncbi.nlm.nih.gov/31784293/.
https://pubmed.ncbi.nlm.nih.gov/25564805/. https://pubmed.ncbi.nlm.nih.gov/38057017/.
https://pubmed.ncbi.nlm.nih.gov/6438480/.

574. Articles: https://pubmed.ncbi.nlm.nih.gov/29064205/.
https://pubmed.ncbi.nlm.nih.gov/22171613/. https://pubmed.ncbi.nlm.nih.gov/25155458/.

575. Articles: https://pubmed.ncbi.nlm.nih.gov/35063189/.
https://pubmed.ncbi.nlm.nih.gov/32229174/. https://pubmed.ncbi.nlm.nih.gov/31611877/.
https://pubmed.ncbi.nlm.nih.gov/36387030/.

576. Article: https://pubmed.ncbi.nlm.nih.gov/46514/.

577. Articles: https://pubmed.ncbi.nlm.nih.gov/33836479/.
https://pubmed.ncbi.nlm.nih.gov/33215701/. https://pubmed.ncbi.nlm.nih.gov/31622132/.
https://pubmed.ncbi.nlm.nih.gov/22672495/.

578. Articles: https://pubmed.ncbi.nlm.nih.gov/32105814/.
https://pubmed.ncbi.nlm.nih.gov/7027768/. https://pubmed.ncbi.nlm.nih.gov/32143624/.
https://pubmed.ncbi.nlm.nih.gov/181342/. https://pubmed.ncbi.nlm.nih.gov/2133956/.

579. Article:
https://www.webmd.com/vitamins-and-supplements/what-to-know-about-vitamin-d-and-mental-health.

580. Articles: https://pubmed.ncbi.nlm.nih.gov/31736391/.
https://pubmed.ncbi.nlm.nih.gov/37874187/.

581. Articles: https://pubmed.ncbi.nlm.nih.gov/11096695/.
https://pubmed.ncbi.nlm.nih.gov/28138903/. https://pubmed.ncbi.nlm.nih.gov/14664769/.
https://pubmed.ncbi.nlm.nih.gov/33577006/. https://pubmed.ncbi.nlm.nih.gov/38169875/.

582. Related articles: https://pubmed.ncbi.nlm.nih.gov/31963460/.
https://pubmed.ncbi.nlm.nih.gov/32241571/. https://pubmed.ncbi.nlm.nih.gov/30019090/.

583. Articles: https://www.healthylife.com.au/learn/chicken-pox.
https://pubmed.ncbi.nlm.nih.gov/25487609/. https://pubmed.ncbi.nlm.nih.gov/38423817/.
https://www.ukbiobank.ac.uk/enable-your-research/approved-research/association-between-serum-vi
tamin-d-deficiency-and-the-risk-of-herpes-zoster-a-longitudinal-uk-biobank-study.

584. Articles: https://pubmed.ncbi.nlm.nih.gov/35063189/.
https://pubmed.ncbi.nlm.nih.gov/32229174/. https://pubmed.ncbi.nlm.nih.gov/31611877/.
https://pubmed.ncbi.nlm.nih.gov/36387030/.

585. Articles: https://pubmed.ncbi.nlm.nih.gov/19814946/.
https://pubmed.ncbi.nlm.nih.gov/28877925/. https://pubmed.ncbi.nlm.nih.gov/32043332/.
https://pubmed.ncbi.nlm.nih.gov/33019891/.

586. Articles: https://pubmed.ncbi.nlm.nih.gov/24516688/.
https://pubmed.ncbi.nlm.nih.gov/32908795/. https://pubmed.ncbi.nlm.nih.gov/34802410/.

587. Articles: https://pubmed.ncbi.nlm.nih.gov/11952079/. Related articles:
https://pubmed.ncbi.nlm.nih.gov/30567100/. https://pubmed.ncbi.nlm.nih.gov/27170613/.

588. Articles: https://pubmed.ncbi.nlm.nih.gov/27097975/.
https://pubmed.ncbi.nlm.nih.gov/20719979/. https://pubmed.ncbi.nlm.nih.gov/35257799/.
https://pubmed.ncbi.nlm.nih.gov/17002932/.

589. Articles: https://pubmed.ncbi.nlm.nih.gov/37866777/.
https://pubmed.ncbi.nlm.nih.gov/28913106/.
https://www.sciencedirect.com/science/article/abs/pii/S2468784723001459#:~:text=Vitamin%20
D%20is%20an%20immunomodulator,status%20associated%20with%20hyperemesis%20gravidarum.

590. Articles: https://www.ncbi.nlm.nih.gov/pmc/articles/PMC4776554/.
https://www.mdpi.com/2813-2998/2/4/46#:~:text=Vitamin%20D%20plays%20a%20crucial,to%2
0elevated%20blood%20glucose%20levels.

591. Articles: https://pubmed.ncbi.nlm.nih.gov/29669433/.
https://pubmed.ncbi.nlm.nih.gov/33738914/.

592. Article: https://pubmed.ncbi.nlm.nih.gov/20301786/.

593. Article: https://pubmed.ncbi.nlm.nih.gov/21258262/. See also Bowles, p. 62.

594. Articles: https://pubmed.ncbi.nlm.nih.gov/25916759/.
https://pubmed.ncbi.nlm.nih.gov/27858283/. https://pubmed.ncbi.nlm.nih.gov/21985980/.
https://pubmed.ncbi.nlm.nih.gov/22544696/. Studies confirm that patients treated with vitamin D
showed improvements. Zaidi, pp. 35-39.

595. Articles: https://pubmed.ncbi.nlm.nih.gov/29112461/.
https://pubmed.ncbi.nlm.nih.gov/38929559/. https://pubmed.ncbi.nlm.nih.gov/37242186/.
https://pubmed.ncbi.nlm.nih.gov/37522690/. https://pubmed.ncbi.nlm.nih.gov/35429802/.
https://pubmed.ncbi.nlm.nih.gov/32649802/.

596. Related article: https://pubmed.ncbi.nlm.nih.gov/38269219/.

597. Articles: https://pubmed.ncbi.nlm.nih.gov/21206551/.
https://pubmed.ncbi.nlm.nih.gov/37965409/. https://pubmed.ncbi.nlm.nih.gov/9539254/.

598. Articles: https://pubmed.ncbi.nlm.nih.gov/29401665/.
https://pubmed.ncbi.nlm.nih.gov/38008680/. https://pubmed.ncbi.nlm.nih.gov/32899880/.

599. Articles: https://pubmed.ncbi.nlm.nih.gov/28895880/.
https://pubmed.ncbi.nlm.nih.gov/35784564/. https://pubmed.ncbi.nlm.nih.gov/35440339/.
https://pubmed.ncbi.nlm.nih.gov/34291533/. https://pubmed.ncbi.nlm.nih.gov/26171622/.
https://pubmed.ncbi.nlm.nih.gov/26680495/.

600. Related articles: https://pubmed.ncbi.nlm.nih.gov/26767392/.
https://pubmed.ncbi.nlm.nih.gov/25311777/. https://pubmed.ncbi.nlm.nih.gov/38292780/.
https://pubmed.ncbi.nlm.nih.gov/24803734/. https://pubmed.ncbi.nlm.nih.gov/23816059/.

601. Article: https://pubmed.ncbi.nlm.nih.gov/33983694/.

602. Articles: https://pubmed.ncbi.nlm.nih.gov/33550962/.
https://pubmed.ncbi.nlm.nih.gov/28483335/. https://pubmed.ncbi.nlm.nih.gov/29172025/.
https://pubmed.ncbi.nlm.nih.gov/24859729/. Some individuals experience reduced problems with
hypoglycemia taking high dosages of vitamin D3. Bowles, pp. 185-186.
603. Articles: https://pubmed.ncbi.nlm.nih.gov/25044703/.
https://pubmed.ncbi.nlm.nih.gov/24238472/. https://pubmed.ncbi.nlm.nih.gov/35498428/.
https://pubmed.ncbi.nlm.nih.gov/37750061/.
604. Articles: https://pubmed.ncbi.nlm.nih.gov/37000405/.
https://pubmed.ncbi.nlm.nih.gov/31116878/. https://pubmed.ncbi.nlm.nih.gov/32555278/.
https://pubmed.ncbi.nlm.nih.gov/33484571/. https://pubmed.ncbi.nlm.nih.gov/35072832/.
https://pubmed.ncbi.nlm.nih.gov/30551988/.
605. Articles: https://pubmed.ncbi.nlm.nih.gov/22319799/.
https://pubmed.ncbi.nlm.nih.gov/38365463/. https://pubmed.ncbi.nlm.nih.gov/37084401/.
https://pubmed.ncbi.nlm.nih.gov/22863286/.
606. Articles: https://pubmed.ncbi.nlm.nih.gov/29368588/.
https://pubmed.ncbi.nlm.nih.gov/29478008/. https://pubmed.ncbi.nlm.nih.gov/34969230/.
https://pubmed.ncbi.nlm.nih.gov/26511949/.
607. Articles: https://pubmed.ncbi.nlm.nih.gov/34628636/.
https://pubmed.ncbi.nlm.nih.gov/34537827/. https://pubmed.ncbi.nlm.nih.gov/32902636/.
https://pubmed.ncbi.nlm.nih.gov/22789765/. https://pubmed.ncbi.nlm.nih.gov/24444004/.
https://pubmed.ncbi.nlm.nih.gov/32554649/.
608. Articles: https://pubmed.ncbi.nlm.nih.gov/28315909/.
https://pubmed.ncbi.nlm.nih.gov/37593614/. https://pubmed.ncbi.nlm.nih.gov/37698908/.
https://pubmed.ncbi.nlm.nih.gov/36299985/. https://pubmed.ncbi.nlm.nih.gov/38239402/.
https://pubmed.ncbi.nlm.nih.gov/32192469/. https://pubmed.ncbi.nlm.nih.gov/35440339/.
609. Articles: https://pubmed.ncbi.nlm.nih.gov/35406562/.
https://pubmed.ncbi.nlm.nih.gov/35711312/. https://pubmed.ncbi.nlm.nih.gov/30514196/.
https://pubmed.ncbi.nlm.nih.gov/34126416/. https://pubmed.ncbi.nlm.nih.gov/32712621/.
https://pubmed.ncbi.nlm.nih.gov/37878884/.
610. Articles: https://pubmed.ncbi.nlm.nih.gov/33396382/.
https://pubmed.ncbi.nlm.nih.gov/37781953/. https://pubmed.ncbi.nlm.nih.gov/29762159/.
https://pubmed.ncbi.nlm.nih.gov/31779998/.
611. Articles: https://pubmed.ncbi.nlm.nih.gov/37214583/.
https://pubmed.ncbi.nlm.nih.gov/37576336/. https://pubmed.ncbi.nlm.nih.gov/37260904/.
https://pubmed.ncbi.nlm.nih.gov/35807798/.
612. Articles: https://pubmed.ncbi.nlm.nih.gov/29169714/.
https://pubmed.ncbi.nlm.nih.gov/33229759/. https://pubmed.ncbi.nlm.nih.gov/26498119/.
https://pubmed.ncbi.nlm.nih.gov/7632510/.
613. Articles: https://pubmed.ncbi.nlm.nih.gov/37612740/.
https://pubmed.ncbi.nlm.nih.gov/34400742/. https://pubmed.ncbi.nlm.nih.gov/36389018/.
https://pubmed.ncbi.nlm.nih.gov/30659895/. https://pubmed.ncbi.nlm.nih.gov/35265706/.
614. Related article: https://www.ncbi.nlm.nih.gov/pmc/articles/PMC9220304/.
615. Articles: https://pubmed.ncbi.nlm.nih.gov/27505106/.
https://www.ncbi.nlm.nih.gov/pmc/articles/PMC6108041/.
https://austinpublishinggroup.com/nutritional-disorders/fulltext/andt-v8-id1068.php#:~:text=Vitami
n%20D%20repletion%20may%20reduce,of%20illness%20in%20infectious%20mononucleosis.
616. Articles: https://pubmed.ncbi.nlm.nih.gov/34322844/.
https://pubmed.ncbi.nlm.nih.gov/32349265/. https://pubmed.ncbi.nlm.nih.gov/36857810/.
https://pubmed.ncbi.nlm.nih.gov/21133662/.
617. Articles: https://pubmed.ncbi.nlm.nih.gov/21527855/.
https://pubmed.ncbi.nlm.nih.gov/37686873/. https://pubmed.ncbi.nlm.nih.gov/23857223/.
https://pubmed.ncbi.nlm.nih.gov/19172691/.
618. Articles: https://pubmed.ncbi.nlm.nih.gov/35963983/.
https://pubmed.ncbi.nlm.nih.gov/26282157/. https://pubmed.ncbi.nlm.nih.gov/37035834/.
https://pubmed.ncbi.nlm.nih.gov/38272820/.
619. Articles: https://pubmed.ncbi.nlm.nih.gov/902841/.
https://pubmed.ncbi.nlm.nih.gov/7095227/. https://pubmed.ncbi.nlm.nih.gov/2994578/.
620. Articles: https://pubmed.ncbi.nlm.nih.gov/34491371/.
https://pubmed.ncbi.nlm.nih.gov/32387293/. https://pubmed.ncbi.nlm.nih.gov/34132863/.
https://pubmed.ncbi.nlm.nih.gov/26979990/.

621. Articles: https://pubmed.ncbi.nlm.nih.gov/37811112/.
https://pubmed.ncbi.nlm.nih.gov/37691106/. https://pubmed.ncbi.nlm.nih.gov/38877334/.
https://pubmed.ncbi.nlm.nih.gov/36994062/.

622. Articles: https://pubmed.ncbi.nlm.nih.gov/34322844/.
https://pubmed.ncbi.nlm.nih.gov/21133662/. https://pubmed.ncbi.nlm.nih.gov/32679784/.
https://pubmed.ncbi.nlm.nih.gov/25881523/.

623. Articles: https://pubmed.ncbi.nlm.nih.gov/27505106/.
https://www.ncbi.nlm.nih.gov/pmc/articles/PMC6108041/.
https://austinpublishinggroup.com/nutritional-disorders/fulltext/andt-v8-id1068.php#:~:text=Vitami
n%20D%20repletion%20may%20reduce,of%20illness%20in%20infectious%20mononucleosis.

624. Articles: https://pubmed.ncbi.nlm.nih.gov/37266579/.
https://pubmed.ncbi.nlm.nih.gov/35526493/. https://pubmed.ncbi.nlm.nih.gov/37299485/.
https://pubmed.ncbi.nlm.nih.gov/34139003/.

625. Articles:https://pubmed.ncbi.nlm.nih.gov/36593707/.
https://pubmed.ncbi.nlm.nih.gov/34289935/. https://pubmed.ncbi.nlm.nih.gov/36741485/.
https://pubmed.ncbi.nlm.nih.gov/34247390/.

626. Articles: https://pubmed.ncbi.nlm.nih.gov/23239393/.
https://pubmed.ncbi.nlm.nih.gov/25048990/. https://pubmed.ncbi.nlm.nih.gov/37379302/.

627. Articles: https://pubmed.ncbi.nlm.nih.gov/33396382/.
https://pubmed.ncbi.nlm.nih.gov/37781953/. https://pubmed.ncbi.nlm.nih.gov/29762159/.
https://pubmed.ncbi.nlm.nih.gov/31779998/.

628. Articles: https://pubmed.ncbi.nlm.nih.gov/33397599/.
https://pubmed.ncbi.nlm.nih.gov/29080634/. https://pubmed.ncbi.nlm.nih.gov/29348609/.

629. Articles: https://pubmed.ncbi.nlm.nih.gov/32252338/.
https://pubmed.ncbi.nlm.nih.gov/34827621/. https://pubmed.ncbi.nlm.nih.gov/22797987/.
https://pubmed.ncbi.nlm.nih.gov/37407993/. https://pubmed.ncbi.nlm.nih.gov/16959053/. See
also Khalsa, pp. 133-135.

630. Articles: https://pubmed.ncbi.nlm.nih.gov/17011719/.
https://pubmed.ncbi.nlm.nih.gov/16563471/. https://pubmed.ncbi.nlm.nih.gov/30591925/.
https://pubmed.ncbi.nlm.nih.gov/30591925/. https://pubmed.ncbi.nlm.nih.gov/34444863/.
https://pubmed.ncbi.nlm.nih.gov/34718967/. https://pubmed.ncbi.nlm.nih.gov/36698822/.

631. Articles: https://pubmed.ncbi.nlm.nih.gov/19383117/.
https://pubmed.ncbi.nlm.nih.gov/22715179/. https://pubmed.ncbi.nlm.nih.gov/26981576/.
https://pubmed.ncbi.nlm.nih.gov/25101194/.

632. Articles:
https://www.nutri-facts.org/en_US/news/articles/vitamin-d-may-help-prevent-ear-infections.html.
https://ejo.springeropen.com/articles/10.1186/s43163-022-00199-w.
https://www.ncbi.nlm.nih.gov/pmc/articles/PMC10657834/. Related:
https://lmhofmeyr.co.za/bppv-low-vitamin-d/.

633. Articles: https://pubmed.ncbi.nlm.nih.gov/31506836/.
https://pubmed.ncbi.nlm.nih.gov/30959886/. https://pubmed.ncbi.nlm.nih.gov/32932777/.

634. Articles: https://pubmed.ncbi.nlm.nih.gov/35163353/.
https://pubmed.ncbi.nlm.nih.gov/32847829/. https://pubmed.ncbi.nlm.nih.gov/34917293/.
https://pubmed.ncbi.nlm.nih.gov/32884728/.

635. Article:
https://www.webmd.com/vitamins-and-supplements/what-to-know-about-vitamin-d-and-mental-healt
h.

636. Article: https://welevelupwa.com/mental-health/intermittent-explosive-disorder/.

637. Related articles: https://pubmed.ncbi.nlm.nih.gov/35682491/.
https://pubmed.ncbi.nlm.nih.gov/32384728/.

638. Articles: https://pubmed.ncbi.nlm.nih.gov/35283578/.
https://pubmed.ncbi.nlm.nih.gov/34408878/. https://pubmed.ncbi.nlm.nih.gov/23409077/.
https://pubmed.ncbi.nlm.nih.gov/25632848/.

639. Articles: https://pubmed.ncbi.nlm.nih.gov/38241458/.
https://pubmed.ncbi.nlm.nih.gov/36034296/. https://pubmed.ncbi.nlm.nih.gov/33145201/.
https://pubmed.ncbi.nlm.nih.gov/34088910/. https://pubmed.ncbi.nlm.nih.gov/38347057/.
https://pubmed.ncbi.nlm.nih.gov/36764983/.

640. Articles: https://pubmed.ncbi.nlm.nih.gov/35482784/.
https://pubmed.ncbi.nlm.nih.gov/29978524/. https://pubmed.ncbi.nlm.nih.gov/2663512/.
https://pubmed.ncbi.nlm.nih.gov/33447990/. https://pubmed.ncbi.nlm.nih.gov/3781071/.
https://pubmed.ncbi.nlm.nih.gov/21986726/. https://pubmed.ncbi.nlm.nih.gov/20955096/.
https://pubmed.ncbi.nlm.nih.gov/230129/.
641. Articles: https://pubmed.ncbi.nlm.nih.gov/38751252/.
https://pubmed.ncbi.nlm.nih.gov/22014374/. https://pubmed.ncbi.nlm.nih.gov/32808447/.
https://pubmed.ncbi.nlm.nih.gov/37108056/. https://pubmed.ncbi.nlm.nih.gov/35449997/.
642. Related articles: https://pubmed.ncbi.nlm.nih.gov/35268051/.
https://pubmed.ncbi.nlm.nih.gov/35578558/. https://pubmed.ncbi.nlm.nih.gov/32156230/.
643. Articles: https://pubmed.ncbi.nlm.nih.gov/37214583/.
https://pubmed.ncbi.nlm.nih.gov/37576336/. https://pubmed.ncbi.nlm.nih.gov/37260904/.
https://pubmed.ncbi.nlm.nih.gov/35807798/.
644. Articles: https://pubmed.ncbi.nlm.nih.gov/30744880/.
https://timesofindia.indiatimes.com/life-style/health-fitness/diet/5-nutritional-deficiencies-linked-to-
mood-swings-and-irritability/photostory/106378375.cms.
645. Article:
https://www.webmd.com/vitamins-and-supplements/what-to-know-about-vitamin-d-and-mental-healt
h.
646. Articles: https://pubmed.ncbi.nlm.nih.gov/32454097/.
https://pubmed.ncbi.nlm.nih.gov/33692290/. https://pubmed.ncbi.nlm.nih.gov/37393836/.
https://pubmed.ncbi.nlm.nih.gov/28063040/. https://pubmed.ncbi.nlm.nih.gov/23409301/.
647. Articles: https://pubmed.ncbi.nlm.nih.gov/37954114/.
https://pubmed.ncbi.nlm.nih.gov/31766576/. https://pubmed.ncbi.nlm.nih.gov/1465567/.
https://pubmed.ncbi.nlm.nih.gov/35595176/. https://pubmed.ncbi.nlm.nih.gov/33919716/.
648. Related article: https://pubmed.ncbi.nlm.nih.gov/34197056/.
649. Article: https://pubmed.ncbi.nlm.nih.gov/15847261/.
650. Articles: https://pubmed.ncbi.nlm.nih.gov/29265106/.
https://pubmed.ncbi.nlm.nih.gov/20301427/. https://pubmed.ncbi.nlm.nih.gov/25538884/.
https://pubmed.ncbi.nlm.nih.gov/33380700/. https://pubmed.ncbi.nlm.nih.gov/28368931/.
651. Articles: https://pubmed.ncbi.nlm.nih.gov/23844448/.
https://pubmed.ncbi.nlm.nih.gov/21328097/. https://pubmed.ncbi.nlm.nih.gov/37208906/.
https://pubmed.ncbi.nlm.nih.gov/26545990/. https://pubmed.ncbi.nlm.nih.gov/1410815/.
652. Articles: https://pubmed.ncbi.nlm.nih.gov/38734328/.
https://pubmed.ncbi.nlm.nih.gov/27484684/. https://pubmed.ncbi.nlm.nih.gov/21067953/.
653. Articles: https://www.healthline.com/health/vitamin-d-and-joint-pain.
https://thehouseclinics.co.uk/learning-hub/vitamin-d-relief-for-joint-and-muscle-pain.
https://www.medicalnewstoday.com/articles/321923.
https://www.ncbi.nlm.nih.gov/pmc/articles/PMC5922228/.
654. Articles: https://pubmed.ncbi.nlm.nih.gov/30855798/.
https://pubmed.ncbi.nlm.nih.gov/21918848/.
655. Articles: https://pubmed.ncbi.nlm.nih.gov/34288623/.
https://pubmed.ncbi.nlm.nih.gov/24769175/. https://pubmed.ncbi.nlm.nih.gov/11050002/.
https://pubmed.ncbi.nlm.nih.gov/31838186/. https://pubmed.ncbi.nlm.nih.gov/22683670/.
https://pubmed.ncbi.nlm.nih.gov/23647513/.
656. Article: https://www.ncbi.nlm.nih.gov/pmc/articles/PMC5740515/.
657. Articles: https://pubmed.ncbi.nlm.nih.gov/35831250/.
https://pubmed.ncbi.nlm.nih.gov/28861112/. https://pubmed.ncbi.nlm.nih.gov/38684993/.
https://pubmed.ncbi.nlm.nih.gov/27974130/. https://pubmed.ncbi.nlm.nih.gov/30808315/.
https://pubmed.ncbi.nlm.nih.gov/25994612/.
658. Articles: https://pubmed.ncbi.nlm.nih.gov/11422310/.
https://pubmed.ncbi.nlm.nih.gov/30430523/. https://pubmed.ncbi.nlm.nih.gov/12007693/.
https://pubmed.ncbi.nlm.nih.gov/8845718/.
659. Articles: https://pubmed.ncbi.nlm.nih.gov/33307795/.
https://pubmed.ncbi.nlm.nih.gov/35098071/. https://pubmed.ncbi.nlm.nih.gov/27786545/.
https://pubmed.ncbi.nlm.nih.gov/38770629/.
660. Articles: https://pubmed.ncbi.nlm.nih.gov/?term=vitamin+d+Kidney+cancer.
https://pubmed.ncbi.nlm.nih.gov/37380191/. https://pubmed.ncbi.nlm.nih.gov/36678292/.

661. Articles: https://pubmed.ncbi.nlm.nih.gov/22544696/.
https://pubmed.ncbi.nlm.nih.gov/28346348/. https://pubmed.ncbi.nlm.nih.gov/20077598/.
https://pubmed.ncbi.nlm.nih.gov/21195932/. See also Holick, pp. 235-236.

662. Articles: https://pubmed.ncbi.nlm.nih.gov/22544696/.
https://pubmed.ncbi.nlm.nih.gov/37421259/.

663. Articles: https://pubmed.ncbi.nlm.nih.gov/32032687/.
https://pubmed.ncbi.nlm.nih.gov/30136085/. https://pubmed.ncbi.nlm.nih.gov/29562593/.
https://pubmed.ncbi.nlm.nih.gov/34959915/. See also Dowd and Stafford, pp. 198-200.

664. Articles: https://pubmed.ncbi.nlm.nih.gov/33116949/.
https://pubmed.ncbi.nlm.nih.gov/36174418/.

665. Articles: https://pubmed.ncbi.nlm.nih.gov/37523972/.
https://pubmed.ncbi.nlm.nih.gov/32150754/. https://pubmed.ncbi.nlm.nih.gov/31777808/.

666. Article: https://www.ncbi.nlm.nih.gov/pmc/articles/PMC5922228/.

667. See Bowles, pp. 38-39.

668. Related articles: https://pubmed.ncbi.nlm.nih.gov/23829926/.
https://pubmed.ncbi.nlm.nih.gov/12140916/. https://pubmed.ncbi.nlm.nih.gov/9253619/.

669. Articles: https://pubmed.ncbi.nlm.nih.gov/32759193/.
https://pubmed.ncbi.nlm.nih.gov/38474817/.
https://www.ncbi.nlm.nih.gov/pmc/articles/PMC8377140/.

670. Lactating women tend to be deficient in vitamin D, passing the deficiency onto their infants. This issue is not caused by an inherent D deficiency in human milk, but rather it is due to the fact that most women today do not get enough vitamin D (from the sun, foods, or supplements). When this problem is corrected, human milk has ample vitamin D, which is transferred to the infant. See Zaidi, pp. 168-169.
Articles: https://pubmed.ncbi.nlm.nih.gov/30322097/.
https://pubmed.ncbi.nlm.nih.gov/37569256/. https://pubmed.ncbi.nlm.nih.gov/33232956/.
https://pubmed.ncbi.nlm.nih.gov/21756132/.
https://pubmed.ncbi.nlm.nih.gov/?term=vitamin+d+lactation.
https://pubmed.ncbi.nlm.nih.gov/18290720/.

671. Articles: https://pubmed.ncbi.nlm.nih.gov/34444743/.
https://pubmed.ncbi.nlm.nih.gov/28738753/. https://pubmed.ncbi.nlm.nih.gov/27642086/.
https://pubmed.ncbi.nlm.nih.gov/37834314/. https://pubmed.ncbi.nlm.nih.gov/33316755/.

672. Articles: https://pubmed.ncbi.nlm.nih.gov/36999719/.
https://pubmed.ncbi.nlm.nih.gov/22213311/. https://pubmed.ncbi.nlm.nih.gov/27812016/.
https://pubmed.ncbi.nlm.nih.gov/21527582/.

673. Articles: https://www.ncbi.nlm.nih.gov/pmc/articles/PMC4021247/.
https://www.e-aair.org/pdf/10.4168/aair.2014.6.3.267.
https://www.ncbi.nlm.nih.gov/pmc/articles/PMC9771342/.
https://pubmed.ncbi.nlm.nih.gov/36550807/. Video:
https://www.youtube.com/watch?v=zCmW5bLcE9s.

674. Articles: https://www.ncbi.nlm.nih.gov/pmc/articles/PMC7774915/.
https://www.medscape.com/viewarticle/755046?form=fpf.
https://pubmed.ncbi.nlm.nih.gov/37661522/. https://pubmed.ncbi.nlm.nih.gov/28772303/.

675. Article: https://pubmed.ncbi.nlm.nih.gov/35852202/.

676. Article: https://pubmed.ncbi.nlm.nih.gov/16495324/.

677. Articles: https://pubmed.ncbi.nlm.nih.gov/34684323/.
https://pubmed.ncbi.nlm.nih.gov/28747485/. https://pubmed.ncbi.nlm.nih.gov/20079764/.

678. Articles: https://pubmed.ncbi.nlm.nih.gov/28413421/.
https://pubmed.ncbi.nlm.nih.gov/33275278/. https://pubmed.ncbi.nlm.nih.gov/26780391/.
https://pubmed.ncbi.nlm.nih.gov/15228497/.

679. Though I could not find definitive studies, it is clear that vitamin D may help prevent or treat Legionnaires' disease. See, for example, article:
https://www.thefoodstatecompany.com/legionnaires-disease.

680. Articles: https://pubmed.ncbi.nlm.nih.gov/37671973/.
https://pubmed.ncbi.nlm.nih.gov/35889808/. https://pubmed.ncbi.nlm.nih.gov/16085411/.
https://pubmed.ncbi.nlm.nih.gov/37499549/.

681. Articles: https://pubmed.ncbi.nlm.nih.gov/27809427/.
https://pubmed.ncbi.nlm.nih.gov/38966781/.

682. Articles: https://pubmed.ncbi.nlm.nih.gov/27267638/.
https://pubmed.ncbi.nlm.nih.gov/20301575/.

683. Some individuals experience increased libido taking high dosages of vitamin D3. Bowles, pp. 186-187. See also articles: https://pubmed.ncbi.nlm.nih.gov/27544743/. https://pubmed.ncbi.nlm.nih.gov/20301509/. https://pubmed.ncbi.nlm.nih.gov/29973697/.
684. Articles: https://pubmed.ncbi.nlm.nih.gov/33091918/. https://www.medrxiv.org/content/10.1101/2024.02.21.24303138v2.full. https://www.researchgate.net/publication/331459586_Evaluation_of_Vitamin_D_Levels_in_Patients _with_Lichen_Planus.
685. Articles: https://pubmed.ncbi.nlm.nih.gov/37123896/. https://pubmed.ncbi.nlm.nih.gov/33301353/. https://pubmed.ncbi.nlm.nih.gov/31877381/. https://pubmed.ncbi.nlm.nih.gov/27611796/.
686. Articles: https://pubmed.ncbi.nlm.nih.gov/28414049/. https://pubmed.ncbi.nlm.nih.gov/35406098/.
687. Articles: https://pubmed.ncbi.nlm.nih.gov/34323062/. https://pubmed.ncbi.nlm.nih.gov/38792387/.
688. Articles: https://www.ncbi.nlm.nih.gov/pmc/articles/PMC2839878/. https://www.ncbi.nlm.nih.gov/pmc/articles/PMC8159757/. https://onlinelibrary.wiley.com/doi/10.1155/2020/2656321.
689. Articles: https://pubmed.ncbi.nlm.nih.gov/38662827/. https://pubmed.ncbi.nlm.nih.gov/35505652/. https://pubmed.ncbi.nlm.nih.gov/32229457/. https://pubmed.ncbi.nlm.nih.gov/36986172/.
690. Articles: https://pubmed.ncbi.nlm.nih.gov/33126575/. https://pubmed.ncbi.nlm.nih.gov/37861098/. https://pubmed.ncbi.nlm.nih.gov/31589177/. https://pubmed.ncbi.nlm.nih.gov/36142636/.
691. Articles: https://pubmed.ncbi.nlm.nih.gov/38822077/. https://pubmed.ncbi.nlm.nih.gov/38662827/. https://pubmed.ncbi.nlm.nih.gov/29657326/. https://pubmed.ncbi.nlm.nih.gov/35505652/.
692. Articles: https://www.ncbi.nlm.nih.gov/pmc/articles/PMC4131122/. https://loeysdietzcanada.org/wp-content/uploads/2022/10/LDSFC_Head-to-Toe-of-LDS-Features.pd f.
693. Articles: https://pubmed.ncbi.nlm.nih.gov/17486364/. https://pubmed.ncbi.nlm.nih.gov/37116013/. https://pubmed.ncbi.nlm.nih.gov/33323421/.
694. Articles: https://pubmed.ncbi.nlm.nih.gov/27887750/. https://www.verywellhealth.com/symptoms-of-vitamin-d-deficiency-7963631.
695. Articles: https://pubmed.ncbi.nlm.nih.gov/36613531/. https://pubmed.ncbi.nlm.nih.gov/28380322/. https://pubmed.ncbi.nlm.nih.gov/23570271/.
696. Articles: https://pubmed.ncbi.nlm.nih.gov/36212121/. https://pubmed.ncbi.nlm.nih.gov/32100652/. https://pubmed.ncbi.nlm.nih.gov/34704712/. https://pubmed.ncbi.nlm.nih.gov/24119149/. https://pubmed.ncbi.nlm.nih.gov/28184307/.
697. Articles: https://pubmed.ncbi.nlm.nih.gov/36940921/. https://pubmed.ncbi.nlm.nih.gov/23511683/. https://pubmed.ncbi.nlm.nih.gov/34751419/. https://pubmed.ncbi.nlm.nih.gov/37800763/. https://pubmed.ncbi.nlm.nih.gov/32209124/.
698. Because it can suppress the growth of cancer cells, vitamin D has been found to be successful in both preventing and treating a myriad of cancers. *Food and Nutrition*, p. 30; see also Zaidi, pp. 106-114. Articles: https://pubmed.ncbi.nlm.nih.gov/33225744/. https://pubmed.ncbi.nlm.nih.gov/25967968/. https://pubmed.ncbi.nlm.nih.gov/22213310/.
699. Articles: https://pubmed.ncbi.nlm.nih.gov/36049670/. https://pubmed.ncbi.nlm.nih.gov/28440468/. https://pubmed.ncbi.nlm.nih.gov/27291304/.
700. Articles: https://pubmed.ncbi.nlm.nih.gov/36258153/. https://pubmed.ncbi.nlm.nih.gov/33768348/. https://pubmed.ncbi.nlm.nih.gov/29055500/.
701. Vitamin D deficiency has been linked to autoimmune-inflammatory diseases like lupus. Because lupus patients must avoid exposure to the sun, adequate vitamin D from other sources is imperative for good health. Weiss, p. 221. Articles: https://pubmed.ncbi.nlm.nih.gov/35648165/. https://pubmed.ncbi.nlm.nih.gov/37189455/. https://pubmed.ncbi.nlm.nih.gov/29108830/.
702. Articles: https://pubmed.ncbi.nlm.nih.gov/17699936/. https://www.globallymealliance.org/blog/lyme-and-vitamin-d. https://www.ncbi.nlm.nih.gov/pmc/articles/PMC3520031/. https://www.rupahealth.com/post/a-functional-medicine-chronic-lyme-disease-protocol.
703. Articles: https://pubmed.ncbi.nlm.nih.gov/30247957/. https://pubmed.ncbi.nlm.nih.gov/24644186/. https://pubmed.ncbi.nlm.nih.gov/20170991/. https://pubmed.ncbi.nlm.nih.gov/31140909/.

704. Articles: https://www.ncbi.nlm.nih.gov/pmc/articles/PMC11063265/.
https://pubmed.ncbi.nlm.nih.gov/23201171/.
https://www.dovepress.com/vitamin-d-and-inflammatory-diseases-peer-reviewed-fulltext-article-JIR.
705. Articles: https://pubmed.ncbi.nlm.nih.gov/37189455/.
https://pubmed.ncbi.nlm.nih.gov/38534347/. https://pubmed.ncbi.nlm.nih.gov/33573146/.
https://pubmed.ncbi.nlm.nih.gov/31915915/. https://pubmed.ncbi.nlm.nih.gov/20924963/.
706. Articles:
https://www.wcrf.org/researchwefund/vitamin-d-lifestyle-bowel-cancer-lynch-syndrome/.
https://www.ncbi.nlm.nih.gov/pmc/articles/PMC8193311/.
https://einsteinmed.edu/features/1360/solving-lynch-syndrome/.
https://www.ncbi.nlm.nih.gov/pmc/articles/PMC3688951/.
707. Articles: https://pubmed.ncbi.nlm.nih.gov/32768420/.
https://pubmed.ncbi.nlm.nih.gov/29027953/. https://pubmed.ncbi.nlm.nih.gov/27111565/.
708. Article: https://pubmed.ncbi.nlm.nih.gov/33126575/.
709. Related articles: https://www.ncbi.nlm.nih.gov/pmc/articles/PMC9220304/.
https://typeset.io/papers/the-pathogenesis-of-cardiac-arrhythmias-in-vitamin-d-303x58hk.
710. Articles: https://pubmed.ncbi.nlm.nih.gov/32063570/.
https://pubmed.ncbi.nlm.nih.gov/36465774/. https://pubmed.ncbi.nlm.nih.gov/27479626/.
https://pubmed.ncbi.nlm.nih.gov/31836995/. https://pubmed.ncbi.nlm.nih.gov/29943744/.
https://pubmed.ncbi.nlm.nih.gov/35156551/.
711. This condition prevents absorption of vitamin D. Articles:
https://www.bumc.bu.edu/camed/2021/05/20/study-finds-new-and-effective-treatment-for-vitamin-d-deficiency/. https://link.springer.com/article/10.1007/s11154-023-09792-7.
712. Articles: https://pubmed.ncbi.nlm.nih.gov/30793054/.
https://pubmed.ncbi.nlm.nih.gov/25596566/. https://pubmed.ncbi.nlm.nih.gov/30772945/.
https://pubmed.ncbi.nlm.nih.gov/35416868/. https://pubmed.ncbi.nlm.nih.gov/25470777/.
713. Article: https://pubmed.ncbi.nlm.nih.gov/33197518/.
714. Articles: https://pubmed.ncbi.nlm.nih.gov/19095601/.
https://pubmed.ncbi.nlm.nih.gov/33133014/.
715. Articles: https://pubmed.ncbi.nlm.nih.gov/34205632/.
https://pubmed.ncbi.nlm.nih.gov/33549368/. https://pubmed.ncbi.nlm.nih.gov/38353502/.
https://pubmed.ncbi.nlm.nih.gov/12789152/. https://pubmed.ncbi.nlm.nih.gov/27691906/.
716. Articles: https://pubmed.ncbi.nlm.nih.gov/25713056/.
https://pubmed.ncbi.nlm.nih.gov/33809478/. https://pubmed.ncbi.nlm.nih.gov/38004146/.
https://pubmed.ncbi.nlm.nih.gov/36839310/.
717. Article: https://www.sciencedirect.com/science/article/pii/S1096719214001607.
https://www.ncbi.nlm.nih.gov/pmc/articles/PMC3671925/.
718. Articles: https://pubmed.ncbi.nlm.nih.gov/34152285/.
https://pubmed.ncbi.nlm.nih.gov/25656438/. https://pubmed.ncbi.nlm.nih.gov/22887731/.
719. Articles: https://pubmed.ncbi.nlm.nih.gov/18928561/.
https://pubmed.ncbi.nlm.nih.gov/19090978/. https://pubmed.ncbi.nlm.nih.gov/21156217/.
https://pubmed.ncbi.nlm.nih.gov/2292594/.
720. Articles: https://pubmed.ncbi.nlm.nih.gov/30500845/.
https://pubmed.ncbi.nlm.nih.gov/22082653/. https://pubmed.ncbi.nlm.nih.gov/36759131/.
https://pubmed.ncbi.nlm.nih.gov/22843095/.
721. Articles: https://pubmed.ncbi.nlm.nih.gov/35852202/.
https://pubmed.ncbi.nlm.nih.gov/38795863/.
722. Medications, such as Dilantin, Phenobarbital, Rifampin, Orlistat, Xenical, Alli, Cholestyramine,
Questran, LoCholest, Prevalite, and steroids, may affect vitamin D absorption therefore increasing the
chances of a deficiency. Zaidi, p. 25.
723. Articles: https://pubmed.ncbi.nlm.nih.gov/32940108/.
https://pubmed.ncbi.nlm.nih.gov/28341008/. https://pubmed.ncbi.nlm.nih.gov/27121284/.
https://pubmed.ncbi.nlm.nih.gov/34544219/. https://pubmed.ncbi.nlm.nih.gov/22187059/.
https://pubmed.ncbi.nlm.nih.gov/22193220/.
724. Articles:
https://www.webmd.com/vitamins-and-supplements/what-to-know-about-vitamin-d-and-mental-health. https://www.ncbi.nlm.nih.gov/pmc/articles/PMC9468237/.
https://www.ncbi.nlm.nih.gov/pmc/articles/PMC2908269/.

725. Articles: https://pubmed.ncbi.nlm.nih.gov/28994020/.
https://pubmed.ncbi.nlm.nih.gov/36580363/. https://pubmed.ncbi.nlm.nih.gov/29249122/.
https://pubmed.ncbi.nlm.nih.gov/31892603/. https://pubmed.ncbi.nlm.nih.gov/21371954/.
https://pubmed.ncbi.nlm.nih.gov/32918212/.

726. Vitamin D has been shown to improve memory loss. Altshul and Hops, p. 286. Articles:
https://pubmed.ncbi.nlm.nih.gov/36820164/. https://pubmed.ncbi.nlm.nih.gov/26836174/.
https://pubmed.ncbi.nlm.nih.gov/29422004/.

727. Articles: https://pubmed.ncbi.nlm.nih.gov/33755501/.
https://pubmed.ncbi.nlm.nih.gov/29857909/. https://pubmed.ncbi.nlm.nih.gov/38529449/.

728. Articles: https://pubmed.ncbi.nlm.nih.gov/29297432/.
https://pubmed.ncbi.nlm.nih.gov/30982131/. https://pubmed.ncbi.nlm.nih.gov/27207494/.
https://pubmed.ncbi.nlm.nih.gov/29856234/.

729. Articles: https://pubmed.ncbi.nlm.nih.gov/25563481/.
https://pubmed.ncbi.nlm.nih.gov/37557090/.

730. Articles: https://pubmed.ncbi.nlm.nih.gov/31093951/.
https://pubmed.ncbi.nlm.nih.gov/33809478/. https://pubmed.ncbi.nlm.nih.gov/35156551/.
https://pubmed.ncbi.nlm.nih.gov/37471089/.
https://www.ncbi.nlm.nih.gov/pmc/articles/PMC3886792/.

731. Articles: https://www.ncbi.nlm.nih.gov/pmc/articles/PMC4511535/.
https://pubmed.ncbi.nlm.nih.gov/33865361/. https://pubmed.ncbi.nlm.nih.gov/28176022/.
https://pubmed.ncbi.nlm.nih.gov/20800506/.

732. Some of the complications and discomforts associated with menopause can be mitigated or eliminated by vitamin D, which helps absorb calcium, and all-important mineral in treating menopausal symptoms. Weiss, pp. 229-230. Articles: https://pubmed.ncbi.nlm.nih.gov/38751288/.
https://pubmed.ncbi.nlm.nih.gov/24993517/. https://pubmed.ncbi.nlm.nih.gov/30115856/.

733. Articles: https://pubmed.ncbi.nlm.nih.gov/29447494/.
https://pubmed.ncbi.nlm.nih.gov/36973702/.

734. Articles: https://pubmed.ncbi.nlm.nih.gov/24564337/.
https://pubmed.ncbi.nlm.nih.gov/19095601/. https://pubmed.ncbi.nlm.nih.gov/33133014/.
https://pubmed.ncbi.nlm.nih.gov/1950982/.

735. Article: https://pubmed.ncbi.nlm.nih.gov/33126575/.

736. Articles: https://pubmed.ncbi.nlm.nih.gov/33802330/.
https://pubmed.ncbi.nlm.nih.gov/36768946/. https://pubmed.ncbi.nlm.nih.gov/25813139/.
https://pubmed.ncbi.nlm.nih.gov/24168438/. See also Dowd and Stafford, pp. 132-133; Holick, pp. 95-98.

737. Related article: https://www.ncbi.nlm.nih.gov/books/NBK1328/.

738. Related article: https://www.mdpi.com/2073-4409/10/8/2007.

739. Articles: https://pubmed.ncbi.nlm.nih.gov/18928561/.
https://pubmed.ncbi.nlm.nih.gov/19090978/. https://pubmed.ncbi.nlm.nih.gov/21156217/.
https://pubmed.ncbi.nlm.nih.gov/2292594/.

740. Article: https://www.ncbi.nlm.nih.gov/pmc/articles/PMC5051481/. Related article:
https://www.jkns.or.kr/journal/view.php?number=798.

741. Articles: https://pubmed.ncbi.nlm.nih.gov/31161313/.
https://pubmed.ncbi.nlm.nih.gov/28795503/. https://pubmed.ncbi.nlm.nih.gov/27749530/.
https://pubmed.ncbi.nlm.nih.gov/29447793/. https://pubmed.ncbi.nlm.nih.gov/23694840/.

742. Articles: https://pubmed.ncbi.nlm.nih.gov/37635492/.
https://pubmed.ncbi.nlm.nih.gov/29971976/. https://pubmed.ncbi.nlm.nih.gov/31377873/.
https://pubmed.ncbi.nlm.nih.gov/34879503/.

743. Related articles: https://pubmed.ncbi.nlm.nih.gov/13292141/.
https://pubmed.ncbi.nlm.nih.gov/20296654/. https://pubmed.ncbi.nlm.nih.gov/14159523/.

744. Articles: https://pubmed.ncbi.nlm.nih.gov/35637024/.
https://pubmed.ncbi.nlm.nih.gov/32443760/.
https://www.nih.gov/news-events/news-releases/insufficient-vitamin-d-linked-miscarriage-among-wo
men-prior-pregnancy-loss.
https://www.birmingham.ac.uk/news/2022/vitamin-d-deficiency-and-miscarriage.
https://www.grassrootshealth.net/blog/two-new-studies-show-higher-risk-miscarriage-lower-vitamin-d/.

745. Article: https://pubmed.ncbi.nlm.nih.gov/25115500/.

746. Article: https://www.webmd.com/vitamins-and-supplements/what-to-know-about-vitamin-d-and-mental-healt h.

747. Articles: https://pubmed.ncbi.nlm.nih.gov/26027439/. https://pubmed.ncbi.nlm.nih.gov/31701847/. https://pubmed.ncbi.nlm.nih.gov/35311615/. https://pubmed.ncbi.nlm.nih.gov/36097104/. https://pubmed.ncbi.nlm.nih.gov/29393662/. https://pubmed.ncbi.nlm.nih.gov/18761297/.

748. Articles: https://pubmed.ncbi.nlm.nih.gov/22372707/. https://pubmed.ncbi.nlm.nih.gov/34264451/. https://www.webmd.com/vitamins-and-supplements/what-to-know-about-vitamin-d-and-mental-healt h. https://www.healthline.com/nutrition/depression-and-vitamin-d. https://www.pharmacytimes.com/view/increased-vitamin-d-intake-can-decrease-symptoms-of-depress ion-anxiety.

749. Article: https://pubmed.ncbi.nlm.nih.gov/36998475/.

750. Article: https://pubmed.ncbi.nlm.nih.gov/25115500/.

751. Articles: https://pubmed.ncbi.nlm.nih.gov/37242229/. https://pubmed.ncbi.nlm.nih.gov/30399574/. https://pubmed.ncbi.nlm.nih.gov/31981799/. https://pubmed.ncbi.nlm.nih.gov/37894739/. https://pubmed.ncbi.nlm.nih.gov/37006074/.

752. Articles: https://www.frontiersin.org/journals/nutrition/articles/10.3389/fnut.2023.1132191/full. https://www.ncbi.nlm.nih.gov/pmc/articles/PMC6230238/. https://www.ncbi.nlm.nih.gov/pmc/articles/PMC10325032/. https://www.ijpsonline.com/articles/impact-of-vitamin-dsub3sub-supplementation-on-recurrent-aphth ous-ulcer-4515.html.

753. Articles: https://pubmed.ncbi.nlm.nih.gov/30246874/. https://pubmed.ncbi.nlm.nih.gov/28978801/. https://pubmed.ncbi.nlm.nih.gov/37447304/. https://pubmed.ncbi.nlm.nih.gov/33159645/.

754. Articles: https://pubmed.ncbi.nlm.nih.gov/28628270/. https://pubmed.ncbi.nlm.nih.gov/34611554/. https://pubmed.ncbi.nlm.nih.gov/36072127/. https://pubmed.ncbi.nlm.nih.gov/1395324/.

755. Articles: https://pubmed.ncbi.nlm.nih.gov/36975461/. https://pubmed.ncbi.nlm.nih.gov/37976630/. https://pubmed.ncbi.nlm.nih.gov/38833040/. https://pubmed.ncbi.nlm.nih.gov/35565770/. https://pubmed.ncbi.nlm.nih.gov/33415920/.

756. Articles: https://pubmed.ncbi.nlm.nih.gov/30246874/. https://pubmed.ncbi.nlm.nih.gov/28978801/. https://pubmed.ncbi.nlm.nih.gov/37447304/. https://pubmed.ncbi.nlm.nih.gov/33159645/.

757. Articles: https://pubmed.ncbi.nlm.nih.gov/28628270/. https://pubmed.ncbi.nlm.nih.gov/34611554/. https://pubmed.ncbi.nlm.nih.gov/36072127/. https://pubmed.ncbi.nlm.nih.gov/1395324/.

758. Articles: https://www.ncbi.nlm.nih.gov/pmc/articles/PMC8675347/. https://pubmed.ncbi.nlm.nih.gov/36759131/. https://pubmed.ncbi.nlm.nih.gov/26294740/. https://www.ncbi.nlm.nih.gov/pmc/articles/PMC8653728/. https://www.termedia.pl/Evaluation-of-efficacy-and-safety-of-intralesional-vitamin-D3-in-comparison-with-intralesional-measles-mumps-and-rubella-MMR-vaccine-in-the-treatment-of-multiple-cutaneous-w arts,56,53952,1,1.html.

759. Article: https://www.ncbi.nlm.nih.gov/pmc/articles/PMC3441857/.

760. Articles: https://pubmed.ncbi.nlm.nih.gov/29963601/. https://pubmed.ncbi.nlm.nih.gov/29345167/. https://pubmed.ncbi.nlm.nih.gov/30935447/.

761. Articles: https://pubmed.ncbi.nlm.nih.gov/36346279/. https://pubmed.ncbi.nlm.nih.gov/28007301/.

762. Articles: https://pubmed.ncbi.nlm.nih.gov/31766576/. https://pubmed.ncbi.nlm.nih.gov/35406137/. https://pubmed.ncbi.nlm.nih.gov/33086536/. https://pubmed.ncbi.nlm.nih.gov/32219739/.

763. Articles: https://www.medicalnewstoday.com/articles/324641#common-causes. https://www.physioinqpenrith.com.au/blog/causes-muscle-twitching#:~:text=Vitamin%20D%20defi ciency%20can%20also,vitamin%20D%20from%20sun%20exposure.

764. Articles: https://pubmed.ncbi.nlm.nih.gov/28341251/. https://www.yalemedicine.org/conditions/vitamin-d-deficiency#:~:text=When%20vitamin%20D%2 0levels%20are,muscle%20pain%2C%20and%20muscle%20weakness. https://my.clevelandclinic.org/health/diseases/15050-vitamin-d-vitamin-d-deficiency.

https://www.ncbi.nlm.nih.gov/pmc/articles/PMC3690793/.
765. Articles: https://pubmed.ncbi.nlm.nih.gov/35893864/.
https://pubmed.ncbi.nlm.nih.gov/23649566/. https://pubmed.ncbi.nlm.nih.gov/29057787/.
766. Articles: https://pubmed.ncbi.nlm.nih.gov/29118054/.
https://pubmed.ncbi.nlm.nih.gov/24726169/. https://pubmed.ncbi.nlm.nih.gov/35467812/.
https://pubmed.ncbi.nlm.nih.gov/17507730/.
767. Articles: https://pubmed.ncbi.nlm.nih.gov/36462625/.
https://pubmed.ncbi.nlm.nih.gov/37538922/. https://pubmed.ncbi.nlm.nih.gov/35796450/.
https://pubmed.ncbi.nlm.nih.gov/26822380/.
768. Articles: https://pubmed.ncbi.nlm.nih.gov/28163832/.
https://pubmed.ncbi.nlm.nih.gov/32612689/. https://pubmed.ncbi.nlm.nih.gov/34717822/.
https://pubmed.ncbi.nlm.nih.gov/36480969/.
769. Articles: https://pubmed.ncbi.nlm.nih.gov/35457041/.
https://pubmed.ncbi.nlm.nih.gov/38368573/#:~:text=Vitamin%20D%2C%20as%20a%20kind,have
%20potential%20relationship%20with%20myopia.
https://iovs.arvojournals.org/article.aspx?articleid=2129027.
https://www.ncbi.nlm.nih.gov/pmc/articles/PMC4901111/. See also Bowles, p. 62.
770. Articles: https://pubmed.ncbi.nlm.nih.gov/6894416/.
https://pubmed.ncbi.nlm.nih.gov/6688053/. https://pubmed.ncbi.nlm.nih.gov/166785/.
771. Articles: https://pubmed.ncbi.nlm.nih.gov/23754696/.
https://pubmed.ncbi.nlm.nih.gov/23809192/. https://pubmed.ncbi.nlm.nih.gov/30963668/.
772. Articles: https://pubmed.ncbi.nlm.nih.gov/37861098/.
https://pubmed.ncbi.nlm.nih.gov/36986172/. https://pubmed.ncbi.nlm.nih.gov/28906453/.
https://pubmed.ncbi.nlm.nih.gov/37742738/.
773. Article: https://community.bulksupplements.com/narcissistic-personality-disorder/.
774. Article: https://community.bulksupplements.com/narcissistic-personality-disorder/.
775. Articles: https://pubmed.ncbi.nlm.nih.gov/28153207/.
https://pubmed.ncbi.nlm.nih.gov/21633708/. https://pubmed.ncbi.nlm.nih.gov/32672533/.
https://pubmed.ncbi.nlm.nih.gov/21206551/. https://pubmed.ncbi.nlm.nih.gov/26543719/.
776. Articles: https://pubmed.ncbi.nlm.nih.gov/11499880/.
https://pubmed.ncbi.nlm.nih.gov/37033241/. https://pubmed.ncbi.nlm.nih.gov/14971661/.
https://pubmed.ncbi.nlm.nih.gov/15111823/.
777. Articles: https://pubmed.ncbi.nlm.nih.gov/33132636/.
https://pubmed.ncbi.nlm.nih.gov/34231046/.
778. Articles: https://pubmed.ncbi.nlm.nih.gov/35457041/.
https://pubmed.ncbi.nlm.nih.gov/38368573/#:~:text=Vitamin%20D%2C%20as%20a%20kind,have
%20potential%20relationship%20with%20myopia.
https://iovs.arvojournals.org/article.aspx?articleid=2129027.
https://www.ncbi.nlm.nih.gov/pmc/articles/PMC4901111/.
779. Articles: https://pubmed.ncbi.nlm.nih.gov/31496497/.
https://pubmed.ncbi.nlm.nih.gov/29447493/.
https://thehouseclinics.co.uk/learning-hub/vitamin-d-relief-for-joint-and-muscle-pain.
780. Articles: https://pubmed.ncbi.nlm.nih.gov/22145469/.
https://pubmed.ncbi.nlm.nih.gov/28285303/. https://pubmed.ncbi.nlm.nih.gov/3389874/.
https://pubmed.ncbi.nlm.nih.gov/23396467/. https://pubmed.ncbi.nlm.nih.gov/24821875/.
781. Articles: https://pubmed.ncbi.nlm.nih.gov/32032687/.
https://pubmed.ncbi.nlm.nih.gov/30136085/. https://pubmed.ncbi.nlm.nih.gov/29562593/.
https://pubmed.ncbi.nlm.nih.gov/34959915/.
782. Articles: https://pubmed.ncbi.nlm.nih.gov/36097104/.
https://montarebehavioralhealth.com/blog/vitamin-d-the-connection-to-depression-and-anxiety/#:~:t
ext=Difficulty%20making%20decisions-,Vitamin%20D%20and%20Anxiety,D%20deficiency%20may%
20increase%20anxiety.
https://www.pharmacytimes.com/view/increased-vitamin-d-intake-can-decrease-symptoms-of-depress
ion-anxiety. https://pubmed.ncbi.nlm.nih.gov/31093951/.
https://pubmed.ncbi.nlm.nih.gov/35806075/.
783. Vitamin D regulates calcium in the blood and calcium is necessary for both nerve impulses and
muscle contractions. Smart Nutrition, p. 41. Articles: https://pubmed.ncbi.nlm.nih.gov/36613531/.
https://pubmed.ncbi.nlm.nih.gov/31142227/. https://pubmed.ncbi.nlm.nih.gov/23744412/.
784. Related articles: https://pubmed.ncbi.nlm.nih.gov/7552213/.
https://pubmed.ncbi.nlm.nih.gov/4109739/.

785. Articles: https://pubmed.ncbi.nlm.nih.gov/37779236/.
https://pubmed.ncbi.nlm.nih.gov/35190818/. https://pubmed.ncbi.nlm.nih.gov/38069206/.
https://pubmed.ncbi.nlm.nih.gov/34827697/. https://pubmed.ncbi.nlm.nih.gov/28077289/.
https://pubmed.ncbi.nlm.nih.gov/29257109/.

786. Articles: https://pubmed.ncbi.nlm.nih.gov/36837874/.
https://pubmed.ncbi.nlm.nih.gov/33066259/. https://pubmed.ncbi.nlm.nih.gov/38141750/.
https://pubmed.ncbi.nlm.nih.gov/35156025/. https://pubmed.ncbi.nlm.nih.gov/23445921/.
https://pubmed.ncbi.nlm.nih.gov/16571643/. https://pubmed.ncbi.nlm.nih.gov/33442176/.

787. Related article: https://pubmed.ncbi.nlm.nih.gov/30120219/.

788. Article:
https://omegaquant.com/can-low-vitamin-d-cause-neuropathy/#:~:text=BLOG%3A%20How%20to
%20Choose%20the,the%20hands%20and%2For%20feet.

789. Articles: https://pubmed.ncbi.nlm.nih.gov/33049684/.
https://pubmed.ncbi.nlm.nih.gov/38022259/. https://pubmed.ncbi.nlm.nih.gov/37686834/.
https://pubmed.ncbi.nlm.nih.gov/22796576/. https://pubmed.ncbi.nlm.nih.gov/36049434/.
https://pubmed.ncbi.nlm.nih.gov/38303529/.

790. Articles: https://pubmed.ncbi.nlm.nih.gov/38167239/.
https://pubmed.ncbi.nlm.nih.gov/35607635/.

791. Related articles: https://pubmed.ncbi.nlm.nih.gov/32151694/.
https://pubmed.ncbi.nlm.nih.gov/36806675/. https://pubmed.ncbi.nlm.nih.gov/21274699/.
https://pubmed.ncbi.nlm.nih.gov/24060611/.

792. Articles: https://pubmed.ncbi.nlm.nih.gov/26583614/.
https://pubmed.ncbi.nlm.nih.gov/26988993/. https://pubmed.ncbi.nlm.nih.gov/27267638/.
https://pubmed.ncbi.nlm.nih.gov/38880379/.

793. Articles: https://pubmed.ncbi.nlm.nih.gov/29624812/.
https://pubmed.ncbi.nlm.nih.gov/24636434/.

794. See Zaidi, pp. 165-166. Articles: https://pubmed.ncbi.nlm.nih.gov/29483547/.
https://pubmed.ncbi.nlm.nih.gov/35011008/.

795. Articles: https://pubmed.ncbi.nlm.nih.gov/33573146/.
https://pubmed.ncbi.nlm.nih.gov/31034511/. https://pubmed.ncbi.nlm.nih.gov/19832043/.
https://pubmed.ncbi.nlm.nih.gov/20924963/.

796. Articles: https://pubmed.ncbi.nlm.nih.gov/2204648/.
https://pubmed.ncbi.nlm.nih.gov/28079559/. https://pubmed.ncbi.nlm.nih.gov/2204648/.
https://pubmed.ncbi.nlm.nih.gov/27035899/. https://pubmed.ncbi.nlm.nih.gov/23888288/.

797. Related article: https://pubmed.ncbi.nlm.nih.gov/25936153/.

798. Articles: https://pubmed.ncbi.nlm.nih.gov/34568104/.
https://pubmed.ncbi.nlm.nih.gov/37508748/. While apparently nightmares can be caused by a vitamin
D deficiency, the reverse is also true: good dreams, or what many people call "pleasant" dreams, seem to
be fostered by ample levels of vitamin D. I myself have experienced this phenomenon. L.S. See
"Dreams."

799. Articles:
https://go.gale.com/ps/i.do?id=GALE%7CA600665928&sid=googleScholar&v=2.1&it=r&linkaccess
=abs&issn=21492247&p=AONE&sw=w&userGroupName=anon%7E910983e1&aty=open-web-entry
#:~:text=Children%20with%20sleep%20terror%20with,among%20children%20with%20sleep%20ter
ror.
https://www.researchgate.net/publication/334054145_Vitamin_D_Levels_in_Children_with_Sleep_
Terror_Analytical_Cross-Sectional_Study.
https://omegaquant.com/the-role-of-vitamins-in-promoting-restful-sleep/.
https://search.trdizin.gov.tr/tr/yayin/detay/320178/vitamin-d-levels-in-children-with-sleep-terror-an
alytical-cross-sectional-study.
https://www.drugs.com/comments/cholecalciferol/for-vitamin-d-deficiency.html?page=2.
https://www.healthcentral.com/condition/night-terrors.

800. Articles: https://pubmed.ncbi.nlm.nih.gov/37861098/.
https://pubmed.ncbi.nlm.nih.gov/36986172/. https://pubmed.ncbi.nlm.nih.gov/28906453/.
https://pubmed.ncbi.nlm.nih.gov/37742738/.

801. Articles: https://pubmed.ncbi.nlm.nih.gov/33132636/.
https://pubmed.ncbi.nlm.nih.gov/34231046/.

802. Articles: https://pubmed.ncbi.nlm.nih.gov/33573146/.
https://pubmed.ncbi.nlm.nih.gov/31034511/. https://pubmed.ncbi.nlm.nih.gov/19832043/.
https://pubmed.ncbi.nlm.nih.gov/20924963/.

803. Articles: https://pubmed.ncbi.nlm.nih.gov/34638299/.
https://pubmed.ncbi.nlm.nih.gov/38138233/. https://pubmed.ncbi.nlm.nih.gov/34631325/.
https://pubmed.ncbi.nlm.nih.gov/37237973/. https://pubmed.ncbi.nlm.nih.gov/25087185/.
https://pubmed.ncbi.nlm.nih.gov/18267352/. https://pubmed.ncbi.nlm.nih.gov/33255834/.
804. Articles: https://pubmed.ncbi.nlm.nih.gov/33446957/.
https://pubmed.ncbi.nlm.nih.gov/34492361/. https://pubmed.ncbi.nlm.nih.gov/14676730/.
805. Article: https://pubmed.ncbi.nlm.nih.gov/31504095/.
806. Articles: https://pubmed.ncbi.nlm.nih.gov/29537299/.
https://pubmed.ncbi.nlm.nih.gov/27619037/. https://pubmed.ncbi.nlm.nih.gov/28648890/.
https://pubmed.ncbi.nlm.nih.gov/28647162/. https://pubmed.ncbi.nlm.nih.gov/22311466/.
807. Articles: https://pubmed.ncbi.nlm.nih.gov/33446957/.
https://pubmed.ncbi.nlm.nih.gov/34492361/. https://pubmed.ncbi.nlm.nih.gov/14676730/.
808. Articles: https://drc.bmj.com/content/7/1/e000690.
https://www.aafoot.com/post/could-numbness-in-feet-be-caused-by-a-vitamin-deficiency-fort-worth-podiatry.
https://omegaquant.com/can-low-vitamin-d-cause-neuropathy/#:~:text=BLOG%3A%20How%20to
%20Choose%20the,the%20hands%20and%2For%20feet.
809. Articles: https://pubmed.ncbi.nlm.nih.gov/28915134/.
https://pubmed.ncbi.nlm.nih.gov/35631190/. https://pubmed.ncbi.nlm.nih.gov/33022267/.
https://pubmed.ncbi.nlm.nih.gov/38777414/.
810. Articles: https://pubmed.ncbi.nlm.nih.gov/34551844/.
https://pubmed.ncbi.nlm.nih.gov/36060722/. https://pubmed.ncbi.nlm.nih.gov/30177398/.
https://pubmed.ncbi.nlm.nih.gov/29168423/. https://pubmed.ncbi.nlm.nih.gov/27388777/.
https://psychcentral.com/blog/does-vitamin-d-deficiency-impact-mental-health#ocd.
811. Articles: https://pubmed.ncbi.nlm.nih.gov/30186518/.
https://pubmed.ncbi.nlm.nih.gov/35163353/. https://pubmed.ncbi.nlm.nih.gov/32156230/.
https://pubmed.ncbi.nlm.nih.gov/37704922/. https://pubmed.ncbi.nlm.nih.gov/35645681/.
https://pubmed.ncbi.nlm.nih.gov/29482804/. https://pubmed.ncbi.nlm.nih.gov/28552071/.
812. Articles: https://pubmed.ncbi.nlm.nih.gov/34551844/.
https://pubmed.ncbi.nlm.nih.gov/36060722/. https://pubmed.ncbi.nlm.nih.gov/30177398/.
https://pubmed.ncbi.nlm.nih.gov/29168423/. https://pubmed.ncbi.nlm.nih.gov/27388777/.
813. Articles: https://pubmed.ncbi.nlm.nih.gov/35457041/.
https://pubmed.ncbi.nlm.nih.gov/35684153/. https://pubmed.ncbi.nlm.nih.gov/30467438/.
https://pubmed.ncbi.nlm.nih.gov/25724179/. https://pubmed.ncbi.nlm.nih.gov/34168925/.
814. Articles: https://pubmed.ncbi.nlm.nih.gov/37606927/.
https://pubmed.ncbi.nlm.nih.gov/29375745/. https://pubmed.ncbi.nlm.nih.gov/25905277/.
https://pubmed.ncbi.nlm.nih.gov/32918214/. https://pubmed.ncbi.nlm.nih.gov/27030602/.
815. Articles: https://www.ncbi.nlm.nih.gov/pmc/articles/PMC3315864/.
https://www.sciencedirect.com/science/article/abs/pii/S155637071100157X.
https://www.cambridge.org/core/journals/journal-of-laryngology-and-otology/article/abs/vitamin-d-and-smell-impairment-a-systematic-literature-review/AEB7BBD23006DF87042802BA73250D41.
816. Articles: https://pubmed.ncbi.nlm.nih.gov/34117054/.
https://pubmed.ncbi.nlm.nih.gov/29331964/. https://pubmed.ncbi.nlm.nih.gov/32583342/.
https://www.massgeneral.org/news/press-release/vitamin-d-deficiency-may-increase-risk-for-addictio
n-to-opioids-and-ultraviolet-rays,
817. Article: https://www.ncbi.nlm.nih.gov/pmc/articles/PMC9587585/.
818. Articles: https://pubmed.ncbi.nlm.nih.gov/36428531/.
https://pubmed.ncbi.nlm.nih.gov/37808408/. https://pubmed.ncbi.nlm.nih.gov/36845785/.
https://pubmed.ncbi.nlm.nih.gov/31942011/. https://pubmed.ncbi.nlm.nih.gov/32584274/.
https://pubmed.ncbi.nlm.nih.gov/38907640/.
819. Articles: https://pubmed.ncbi.nlm.nih.gov/26860322/.
https://pubmed.ncbi.nlm.nih.gov/34821593/. https://pubmed.ncbi.nlm.nih.gov/31940621/.
https://pubmed.ncbi.nlm.nih.gov/32996671/.
820. Articles: https://pubmed.ncbi.nlm.nih.gov/32996671/.
https://pubmed.ncbi.nlm.nih.gov/36200993/. https://pubmed.ncbi.nlm.nih.gov/29922939/.
https://pubmed.ncbi.nlm.nih.gov/35218642/.
821. Articles: https://pubmed.ncbi.nlm.nih.gov/26860322/.
https://pubmed.ncbi.nlm.nih.gov/24081895/. https://pubmed.ncbi.nlm.nih.gov/33962013/.
https://pubmed.ncbi.nlm.nih.gov/38373939/. https://pubmed.ncbi.nlm.nih.gov/37810154/.

822. Some studies link a vitamin D deficiency with loss of bone strength. *God-Given Remedies*, p. 272. See also Dowd and Stafford, pp. 183-185. Articles: https://pubmed.ncbi.nlm.nih.gov/36287325/. https://pubmed.ncbi.nlm.nih.gov/28680892/. https://pubmed.ncbi.nlm.nih.gov/30678273/. https://pubmed.ncbi.nlm.nih.gov/33147632/.

823. Related article: https://pubmed.ncbi.nlm.nih.gov/2168944/. https://radiopaedia.org/search?lang=gb&q=osteochondrodysplasia.

824. Articles: https://pubmed.ncbi.nlm.nih.gov/37242473/. https://pubmed.ncbi.nlm.nih.gov/37298368/. https://pubmed.ncbi.nlm.nih.gov/23752159/.

825. Osteomalacia is defined as pain in the ribs, shoulders, spine, pelvis, legs, brittle bones, etc., of adults. See also Frozen shoulder. L.S. Articles: https://pubmed.ncbi.nlm.nih.gov/30321335/. https://pubmed.ncbi.nlm.nih.gov/6387576/. https://pubmed.ncbi.nlm.nih.gov/33390486/. https://pubmed.ncbi.nlm.nih.gov/7014108/. See also Khalsa, pp. 112-113.

826. Articles: https://pubmed.ncbi.nlm.nih.gov/21234807/. https://pubmed.ncbi.nlm.nih.gov/30850084/. https://pubmed.ncbi.nlm.nih.gov/36724911/.

827. This condition is strongly associated with an inadequate intake of vitamin D and calcium. Weiss, p. 264. Affects 25 million Americans. Can be corrected, or at least managed, with the proper balance of vitamin D and calcium. *Smart Nutrition*, pp.274-275. Articles: https://pubmed.ncbi.nlm.nih.gov/26510847/. https://pubmed.ncbi.nlm.nih.gov/24119980/. https://pubmed.ncbi.nlm.nih.gov/18020534/. https://pubmed.ncbi.nlm.nih.gov/11285990/.

828. Articles: https://pubmed.ncbi.nlm.nih.gov/37054849/. https://pubmed.ncbi.nlm.nih.gov/37228489/. https://pubmed.ncbi.nlm.nih.gov/36711643/. https://pubmed.ncbi.nlm.nih.gov/32955002/. https://pubmed.ncbi.nlm.nih.gov/30568875/. https://pubmed.ncbi.nlm.nih.gov/11358669/.

829. Articles: https://www.nutri-facts.org/en_US/news/articles/vitamin-d-may-help-prevent-ear-infections.html. https://ejo.springeropen.com/articles/10.1186/s43163-022-00199-w. https://www.ncbi.nlm.nih.gov/pmc/articles/PMC10657834/. Related: https://lmhofmeyr.co.za/bppv-low-vitamin-d/.

830. Articles: https://pubmed.ncbi.nlm.nih.gov/31161313/. https://pubmed.ncbi.nlm.nih.gov/28795503/. https://pubmed.ncbi.nlm.nih.gov/27749530/. https://pubmed.ncbi.nlm.nih.gov/29447793/. https://pubmed.ncbi.nlm.nih.gov/23694840/.

831. Articles: https://pubmed.ncbi.nlm.nih.gov/17907013/. https://ejo.springeropen.com/articles/10.1186/s43163-022-00199-w. https://www.nutri-facts.org/en_US/news/articles/vitamin-d-may-help-prevent-ear-infections.html.

832. Articles: https://pubmed.ncbi.nlm.nih.gov/23639864/. https://pubmed.ncbi.nlm.nih.gov/3927224/. https://pubmed.ncbi.nlm.nih.gov/6602194/. https://pubmed.ncbi.nlm.nih.gov/26656733/.

833. Articles: https://pubmed.ncbi.nlm.nih.gov/17907013/. https://ejo.springeropen.com/articles/10.1186/s43163-022-00199-w. https://www.nutri-facts.org/en_US/news/articles/vitamin-d-may-help-prevent-ear-infections.html.

834. Articles: https://pubmed.ncbi.nlm.nih.gov/32059597/. https://pubmed.ncbi.nlm.nih.gov/30041759/. https://pubmed.ncbi.nlm.nih.gov/36145244/. https://pubmed.ncbi.nlm.nih.gov/24870722/. https://pubmed.ncbi.nlm.nih.gov/32814859/. https://pubmed.ncbi.nlm.nih.gov/21324518/.

835. Articles: https://pubmed.ncbi.nlm.nih.gov/37266579/. https://pubmed.ncbi.nlm.nih.gov/35458211/. https://pubmed.ncbi.nlm.nih.gov/24933120/. https://pubmed.ncbi.nlm.nih.gov/32481491/. https://pubmed.ncbi.nlm.nih.gov/31187648/. https://pubmed.ncbi.nlm.nih.gov/30665436/.

836. Articles: https://pubmed.ncbi.nlm.nih.gov/28895880/. https://pubmed.ncbi.nlm.nih.gov/32545596/. https://pubmed.ncbi.nlm.nih.gov/35440339/. https://pubmed.ncbi.nlm.nih.gov/26680495/. https://pubmed.ncbi.nlm.nih.gov/25514898/. https://pubmed.ncbi.nlm.nih.gov/32666762/. https://pubmed.ncbi.nlm.nih.gov/35784564/.

837. Articles: https://pubmed.ncbi.nlm.nih.gov/32353565/. https://pubmed.ncbi.nlm.nih.gov/31236621/. https://pubmed.ncbi.nlm.nih.gov/31634910/. https://pubmed.ncbi.nlm.nih.gov/24232814/. https://pubmed.ncbi.nlm.nih.gov/24365358/. https://pubmed.ncbi.nlm.nih.gov/27068613/. https://pubmed.ncbi.nlm.nih.gov/22307369/.

838. Article: https://pubmed.ncbi.nlm.nih.gov/29057787/.

839. Articles: https://academic.oup.com/painmedicine/article/15/9/1609/1894292. https://pubmed.ncbi.nlm.nih.gov/24730754/. https://www.yalemedicine.org/conditions/vitamin-d-deficiency.

840. Articles:
https://www.asarchcenter.com/blog/which-vitamin-deficiency-causes-white-spots-on-skin/.
https://timesofindia.indiatimes.com/life-style/health-fitness/health-news/vitamin-d-deficiency-look-fo
r-these-5-signs-on-your-skin/photostory/106897203.cms.
841. Articles: https://pubmed.ncbi.nlm.nih.gov/26276715/.
https://pubmed.ncbi.nlm.nih.gov/34072725/. https://pubmed.ncbi.nlm.nih.gov/25259922/. See
also Zaidi, pp. 106-114.
842. Articles: https://pubmed.ncbi.nlm.nih.gov/35631254/.
https://pubmed.ncbi.nlm.nih.gov/30788120/. https://pubmed.ncbi.nlm.nih.gov/27453461/.
https://pubmed.ncbi.nlm.nih.gov/28029611/. https://pubmed.ncbi.nlm.nih.gov/25259922/.
843. Articles: https://pubmed.ncbi.nlm.nih.gov/32109855/.
https://pubmed.ncbi.nlm.nih.gov/23395104/. https://pubmed.ncbi.nlm.nih.gov/37054418/.
https://pubmed.ncbi.nlm.nih.gov/37204025/.
844. Articles: https://pubmed.ncbi.nlm.nih.gov/25905214/.
https://pubmed.ncbi.nlm.nih.gov/28703535/. https://pubmed.ncbi.nlm.nih.gov/29915661/.
845. Articles: https://pubmed.ncbi.nlm.nih.gov/32301688/.
https://pubmed.ncbi.nlm.nih.gov/37091462/. https://pubmed.ncbi.nlm.nih.gov/37875632/.
846. Related articles: https://pubmed.ncbi.nlm.nih.gov/36511653/.
https://pubmed.ncbi.nlm.nih.gov/30775554/. https://pubmed.ncbi.nlm.nih.gov/32504138/.
https://pubmed.ncbi.nlm.nih.gov/29021995/.
847. Related articles:
https://mosaicdx.com/resource/the-effect-of-vitamin-d-on-psychosis-and-schizophrenia/#:~:text=Th
ose%20with%20vitamin%20D%20deficiency,et%20al.%2C%202012).
https://www.ncbi.nlm.nih.gov/pmc/articles/PMC7322580/.
848. Related articles: https://pubmed.ncbi.nlm.nih.gov/6182580/.
https://www.cambridge.org/core/services/aop-cambridge-core/content/view/91D7538427E080B9B
C91A6125A561CE2/S0924933823022320a.pdf/relation-between-negative-symptoms-and-core-stabilit
y-as-an-indicator-of-functional-exercise-capacity-in-schizophrenia.pdf.
https://pubmed.ncbi.nlm.nih.gov/2740461/.
849. Articles: https://pubmed.ncbi.nlm.nih.gov/27915988/.
https://pubmed.ncbi.nlm.nih.gov/26046559/. https://pubmed.ncbi.nlm.nih.gov/36736658/.
https://www.proceedings.bas.bg/index.php/cr/article/view/412.
https://www.frontiersin.org/journals/cellular-and-infection-microbiology/articles/10.3389/fcimb.20
19.00088/full.
850. Related articles: https://pubmed.ncbi.nlm.nih.gov/35489873/.
https://pubmed.ncbi.nlm.nih.gov/31495905/. https://pubmed.ncbi.nlm.nih.gov/30921001/.
https://pubmed.ncbi.nlm.nih.gov/37694586/. https://pubmed.ncbi.nlm.nih.gov/31427650/.
https://pubmed.ncbi.nlm.nih.gov/38104244/. https://pubmed.ncbi.nlm.nih.gov/36591342/.
851. Articles: https://pubmed.ncbi.nlm.nih.gov/35334877/.
https://pubmed.ncbi.nlm.nih.gov/36613531/. https://pubmed.ncbi.nlm.nih.gov/35741675/.
852. Articles: https://www.ncbi.nlm.nih.gov/pmc/articles/PMC8675347/.
https://pubmed.ncbi.nlm.nih.gov/36759131/. https://pubmed.ncbi.nlm.nih.gov/26294740/.
https://www.ncbi.nlm.nih.gov/pmc/articles/PMC8653728/.
https://www.termedia.pl/Evaluation-of-efficacy-and-safety-of-intralesional-vitamin-D3-in-comparison-
with-intralesional-measles-mumps-and-rubella-MMR-vaccine-in-the-treatment-of-multiple-cutaneous-w
arts,56,53952,1,1.html.
853. Article: https://maze.conductscience.com/vitamin-d-and-anxiety/.
854. Articles:
https://journalofsportsmedicine.org/abstract/361/eng#:~:text=Results%3A%20Serum%2025%2Dhy
droxyvitamin%20D,26.9%C2%B110.6%20ng%2Fml.
https://www.ncbi.nlm.nih.gov/pmc/articles/PMC8167354/.
https://journals.sagepub.com/doi/10.1177/19417381231172726?icid=int.sj-full-text.citing-articles.8.
Related: https://pubmed.ncbi.nlm.nih.gov/14563459/.
https://pubmed.ncbi.nlm.nih.gov/33301353/. https://pubmed.ncbi.nlm.nih.gov/38795863/.
855. Articles: https://pubmed.ncbi.nlm.nih.gov/31576965/.
https://pubmed.ncbi.nlm.nih.gov/35458211/. https://pubmed.ncbi.nlm.nih.gov/36479481/.
https://pubmed.ncbi.nlm.nih.gov/34293835/. https://pubmed.ncbi.nlm.nih.gov/36427990/.
https://pubmed.ncbi.nlm.nih.gov/37427232/.

856. Articles: https://pubmed.ncbi.nlm.nih.gov/34288623/.
https://pubmed.ncbi.nlm.nih.gov/26666941/. https://pubmed.ncbi.nlm.nih.gov/28760906/.
https://pubmed.ncbi.nlm.nih.gov/19857741/. https://pubmed.ncbi.nlm.nih.gov/30892756/.
https://pubmed.ncbi.nlm.nih.gov/38874038/.

857. Related article: https://www.ncbi.nlm.nih.gov/pmc/articles/PMC7417489/.

858. Articles: https://pubmed.ncbi.nlm.nih.gov/33977890/.
https://pubmed.ncbi.nlm.nih.gov/34349978/. https://pubmed.ncbi.nlm.nih.gov/36620233/.
https://pubmed.ncbi.nlm.nih.gov/35016636/. Related:
https://pubmed.ncbi.nlm.nih.gov/28083018/.

859. Article: https://pubmed.ncbi.nlm.nih.gov/26882809/.

860. Articles: https://pubmed.ncbi.nlm.nih.gov/35927747/.
https://pubmed.ncbi.nlm.nih.gov/37777909/. https://pubmed.ncbi.nlm.nih.gov/37633644/.
https://pubmed.ncbi.nlm.nih.gov/26167056/. https://pubmed.ncbi.nlm.nih.gov/20308841/.

861. Related article: https://pubmed.ncbi.nlm.nih.gov/17200157/.

862. Some studies have shown that vitamin D reduces cancer and cancer risks wherever it appears in the body. See article: https://pubmed.ncbi.nlm.nih.gov/17721433/. Related articles:
https://onlinelibrary.wiley.com/doi/10.1155/2018/6030646.
https://www.ncbi.nlm.nih.gov/pmc/articles/PMC7752519/.

863. Related articles: https://pubmed.ncbi.nlm.nih.gov/29055500/.
https://pubmed.ncbi.nlm.nih.gov/29442458/. https://pubmed.ncbi.nlm.nih.gov/21012744/.
https://pubmed.ncbi.nlm.nih.gov/2253823/. https://pubmed.ncbi.nlm.nih.gov/24060611/.
https://pubmed.ncbi.nlm.nih.gov/1763670/.

864. Articles: https://pubmed.ncbi.nlm.nih.gov/24746456/.
https://pubmed.ncbi.nlm.nih.gov/30870794/.

865. A balanced program of vitamin D, calcium, and phosphorus seems to lead to improvements in dental health. Hausman and Hurley, p. 171. Articles: https://pubmed.ncbi.nlm.nih.gov/32438644/.
https://pubmed.ncbi.nlm.nih.gov/36537578/. https://pubmed.ncbi.nlm.nih.gov/31199730/.
https://pubmed.ncbi.nlm.nih.gov/36048921/.

866. Articles: https://pubmed.ncbi.nlm.nih.gov/28516265/.
https://pubmed.ncbi.nlm.nih.gov/32708032/. https://pubmed.ncbi.nlm.nih.gov/35112385/.
https://pubmed.ncbi.nlm.nih.gov/33809193/. https://pubmed.ncbi.nlm.nih.gov/30364037/.
https://pubmed.ncbi.nlm.nih.gov/38541146/. https://pubmed.ncbi.nlm.nih.gov/38096511/.

867. Dark circles under the eyes. Bowles, p. 189.

868. Articles: https://pubmed.ncbi.nlm.nih.gov/31623356/.
https://pubmed.ncbi.nlm.nih.gov/22140318/. https://pubmed.ncbi.nlm.nih.gov/32520144/.
https://pubmed.ncbi.nlm.nih.gov/20511096/. https://pubmed.ncbi.nlm.nih.gov/22835416/.

869. Articles: https://pubmed.ncbi.nlm.nih.gov/35428527/.
https://pubmed.ncbi.nlm.nih.gov/37337761/. https://pubmed.ncbi.nlm.nih.gov/30102801/.
https://omegaquant.com/can-low-vitamin-d-cause-neuropathy/#:~:text=BLOG%3A%20How%20to
%20Choose%20the,the%20hands%20and%2For%20feet.

870. Articles: https://pubmed.ncbi.nlm.nih.gov/19669759/.
https://www.mdpi.com/2072-6643/15/21/4571. https://pubmed.ncbi.nlm.nih.gov/14528100/.
https://pubmed.ncbi.nlm.nih.gov/22806259/.
https://www.cancertherapyadvisor.com/news/vitamin-d-supplementation-recommended-for-pediatric
-patients-with-sarcoma/. https://www.ncbi.nlm.nih.gov/pmc/articles/PMC9313306/.
https://www.oncologynurseadvisor.com/news/vitamin-d-supplementation-is-recommended-for-use-in
-young-patients-with-sarcoma/.

871. Articles: https://pubmed.ncbi.nlm.nih.gov/23885887/.
https://pubmed.ncbi.nlm.nih.gov/15492599/. https://pubmed.ncbi.nlm.nih.gov/1320549/.

872. Articles: https://pubmed.ncbi.nlm.nih.gov/26799636/.
https://pubmed.ncbi.nlm.nih.gov/12475388/. https://pubmed.ncbi.nlm.nih.gov/26870934/.
https://pubmed.ncbi.nlm.nih.gov/14713235/.

873. Articles: https://foodforthebrain.org/bpd/. https://pubmed.ncbi.nlm.nih.gov/21274699/.
https://pubmed.ncbi.nlm.nih.gov/31488730/. https://pubmed.ncbi.nlm.nih.gov/32151694/.
https://pubmed.ncbi.nlm.nih.gov/25084800/.
https://www.webmd.com/vitamins-and-supplements/what-to-know-about-vitamin-d-and-mental-healt
h. https://www.ncbi.nlm.nih.gov/pmc/articles/PMC8584834/.

874. Articles: https://pubmed.ncbi.nlm.nih.gov/38008755/.
https://pubmed.ncbi.nlm.nih.gov/36044140/. https://pubmed.ncbi.nlm.nih.gov/37702693/.
https://pubmed.ncbi.nlm.nih.gov/23833127/.

875. Article:
https://www.researchgate.net/publication/269627734_Peutz_Jegher_syndrome_with_multiple_endo
crinal_failures.

876. Articles: https://pubmed.ncbi.nlm.nih.gov/28786261/.
https://pubmed.ncbi.nlm.nih.gov/36742791/. https://pubmed.ncbi.nlm.nih.gov/23246421/.
https://pubmed.ncbi.nlm.nih.gov/37870706/.

877. Articles: https://pubmed.ncbi.nlm.nih.gov/24746456/.
https://pubmed.ncbi.nlm.nih.gov/25009977/.

878. Articles: https://pubmed.ncbi.nlm.nih.gov/29433755/.
https://pubmed.ncbi.nlm.nih.gov/32479158/. https://pubmed.ncbi.nlm.nih.gov/38791104/.
https://pubmed.ncbi.nlm.nih.gov/26835392/. https://pubmed.ncbi.nlm.nih.gov/18394115/.
https://pubmed.ncbi.nlm.nih.gov/24094552/. https://pubmed.ncbi.nlm.nih.gov/25758373/.

879. Articles:
https://www.nutri-facts.org/en_US/news/articles/an-insufficient-vitamin-d-supply-may-be-related-to
-vein-thrombos.html. https://www.ncbi.nlm.nih.gov/pmc/articles/PMC4069050/.
https://us.supersmart.com/en/blog/cardiovascular/phlebitis-what-to-eat-what-not-to-eat-s626.

880. Related articles: https://pubmed.ncbi.nlm.nih.gov/28477263/.
https://pubmed.ncbi.nlm.nih.gov/35895040/.

881. Articles: https://pubmed.ncbi.nlm.nih.gov/38577659/.
https://pubmed.ncbi.nlm.nih.gov/38642359/. https://pubmed.ncbi.nlm.nih.gov/12416085/.
https://pubmed.ncbi.nlm.nih.gov/34522473/.

882. Articles: https://pubmed.ncbi.nlm.nih.gov/30811162/.
https://www.ncbi.nlm.nih.gov/pmc/articles/PMC4192075/.
https://www.aafp.org/pubs/afp/issues/2019/0301/p285.html.

883. Articles:
https://www.sciencedirect.com/topics/nursing-and-health-professions/pilomatrixoma#:~:text=Vita
min%20D%2C%20Calcium%2C%20and%20the,CTNNB1%20overexpression%20to%20induce%20tric
hofolliculomas. https://www.ncbi.nlm.nih.gov/pmc/articles/PMC5348337/.
https://academic.oup.com/bjd/article-abstract/155/1/208/6636960?redirectedFrom=fulltext.

884. Articles: https://pubmed.ncbi.nlm.nih.gov/33977890/.
https://pubmed.ncbi.nlm.nih.gov/34349978/. https://pubmed.ncbi.nlm.nih.gov/36620233/.
https://pubmed.ncbi.nlm.nih.gov/35016636/. Related:
https://pubmed.ncbi.nlm.nih.gov/28083018/.

885. Articles: https://pubmed.ncbi.nlm.nih.gov/23890557/.
https://pubmed.ncbi.nlm.nih.gov/31760824/. https://pubmed.ncbi.nlm.nih.gov/28749078/.
https://pubmed.ncbi.nlm.nih.gov/34319956/. https://pubmed.ncbi.nlm.nih.gov/2454281/.
https://pubmed.ncbi.nlm.nih.gov/37002004/,

886. Articles: https://pubmed.ncbi.nlm.nih.gov/23890557/.
https://pubmed.ncbi.nlm.nih.gov/31760824/. https://pubmed.ncbi.nlm.nih.gov/28749078/.
https://pubmed.ncbi.nlm.nih.gov/34319956/. https://pubmed.ncbi.nlm.nih.gov/2454281/.
https://pubmed.ncbi.nlm.nih.gov/37002004/,

887. Articles: https://pubmed.ncbi.nlm.nih.gov/13584272/.
https://pubmed.ncbi.nlm.nih.gov/15906551/.

888. Articles: https://pubmed.ncbi.nlm.nih.gov/1911337/.
https://www.sciencedirect.com/topics/medicine-and-dentistry/pityriasis-rubra-pilaris.

889. Articles: https://www.bmj.com/rapid-response/2011/11/02/frustrations-vitamin-d-treatments.
https://www.consumerlab.com/answers/supplements-for-plantar-fasciitis-heel-pain/plantar-fasciitis/.
https://www.ncbi.nlm.nih.gov/pmc/articles/PMC2858539/#:~:text=Vitamin%20D%20deficiency%
20commonly%20presents,D%20deficiency%20should%20be%20suspected.

890. Related articles: https://pubmed.ncbi.nlm.nih.gov/32246668/.
https://pubmed.ncbi.nlm.nih.gov/26452590/.

891. Articles; https://pubmed.ncbi.nlm.nih.gov/32162438/.
https://pubmed.ncbi.nlm.nih.gov/32892493/. https://pubmed.ncbi.nlm.nih.gov/31225688/.

892. Articles: https://pubmed.ncbi.nlm.nih.gov/38982373/.
https://pubmed.ncbi.nlm.nih.gov/37950553/.
https://www.ncbi.nlm.nih.gov/pmc/articles/PMC2759054/.

893. Article: https://pubmed.ncbi.nlm.nih.gov/37501941/.

894. Vitamin D has been show to ease the symptoms of PMS. Altshul and Hops, p. 290. Articles:
https://pubmed.ncbi.nlm.nih.gov/29447494/. https://pubmed.ncbi.nlm.nih.gov/30918875/.
https://pubmed.ncbi.nlm.nih.gov/35065636/. https://pubmed.ncbi.nlm.nih.gov/38220382/.

895. Articles: https://pubmed.ncbi.nlm.nih.gov/35428527/.
https://pubmed.ncbi.nlm.nih.gov/37337761/. https://pubmed.ncbi.nlm.nih.gov/30102801/.
https://omegaquant.com/can-low-vitamin-d-cause-neuropathy/#:~:text=BLOG%3A%20How%20to
%20Choose%20the,the%20hands%20and%2For%20feet.
896. Articles: https://pubmed.ncbi.nlm.nih.gov/34288623/.
https://pubmed.ncbi.nlm.nih.gov/26666941/. https://pubmed.ncbi.nlm.nih.gov/28760906/.
https://pubmed.ncbi.nlm.nih.gov/19857741/. https://pubmed.ncbi.nlm.nih.gov/30892756/.
https://pubmed.ncbi.nlm.nih.gov/38874038/.
897. Articles: https://pubmed.ncbi.nlm.nih.gov/32679784/.
https://pubmed.ncbi.nlm.nih.gov/34322844/. https://pubmed.ncbi.nlm.nih.gov/36633175/.
https://pubmed.ncbi.nlm.nih.gov/35507293/. https://pubmed.ncbi.nlm.nih.gov/30024634/.
https://pubmed.ncbi.nlm.nih.gov/34242372/. https://pubmed.ncbi.nlm.nih.gov/32252338/.
898. Dark circles under the eyes. Bowles, p. 189.
899. Articles: https://www.polioplace.org/sites/default/files/files/PPH27-3p1plus.pdf.
https://www.mdpi.com/2076-393X/12/2/121. https://pubmed.ncbi.nlm.nih.gov/38400105/.
https://journals.sagepub.com/doi/abs/10.3181/00379727-48-13353?journalCode=ebma.
900. Articles: https://pubmed.ncbi.nlm.nih.gov/18137144/.
https://pubmed.ncbi.nlm.nih.gov/37853875/. https://pubmed.ncbi.nlm.nih.gov/1217818/.
https://pubmed.ncbi.nlm.nih.gov/2764687/.
901. Articles: https://pubmed.ncbi.nlm.nih.gov/32158346/.
https://pubmed.ncbi.nlm.nih.gov/22086864/. https://pubmed.ncbi.nlm.nih.gov/8182985/.
902. Articles: https://pubmed.ncbi.nlm.nih.gov/23804446/.
https://pubmed.ncbi.nlm.nih.gov/31179282/. https://pubmed.ncbi.nlm.nih.gov/23698116/.
https://pubmed.ncbi.nlm.nih.gov/34821697/.
903. Related article: https://pubmed.ncbi.nlm.nih.gov/28776742/.
904. Articles: https://pubmed.ncbi.nlm.nih.gov/31576965/.
https://pubmed.ncbi.nlm.nih.gov/35458211/. https://pubmed.ncbi.nlm.nih.gov/36479481/.
https://pubmed.ncbi.nlm.nih.gov/34293835/. https://pubmed.ncbi.nlm.nih.gov/36427990/.
https://pubmed.ncbi.nlm.nih.gov/37427232/.
905. Articles: https://pubmed.ncbi.nlm.nih.gov/33577006/.
https://pubmed.ncbi.nlm.nih.gov/35082139/. https://pubmed.ncbi.nlm.nih.gov/31323357/.
https://pubmed.ncbi.nlm.nih.gov/36627860/. https://pubmed.ncbi.nlm.nih.gov/25946084/.
906. Has been to shown to slow with a diet rich in vitamin D. Weiss, p. 229. Articles:
https://pubmed.ncbi.nlm.nih.gov/12520516/. https://pubmed.ncbi.nlm.nih.gov/37937050/.
https://pubmed.ncbi.nlm.nih.gov/34072655/.
907. Articles: https://pubmed.ncbi.nlm.nih.gov/29393662/.
https://pubmed.ncbi.nlm.nih.gov/29649128/. https://pubmed.ncbi.nlm.nih.gov/30657106/.
https://pubmed.ncbi.nlm.nih.gov/34860917/.
908. Articles: https://pubmed.ncbi.nlm.nih.gov/31518608/.
https://pubmed.ncbi.nlm.nih.gov/37685345/.
https://www.sciencedirect.com/science/article/abs/pii/S0278584619305184#:~:text=PTSD%20is
%20associated%20with%20reduced,adjusting%20for%20vitamin%20D%20levels.
https://pubmed.ncbi.nlm.nih.gov/24604440/.
https://www.drjonslaughter.com/post/the-benefits-of-vitamin-d-in-depression-and-ptsd.
https://www.mdpi.com/2075-4418/13/17/2807.
909. Articles: https://pubmed.ncbi.nlm.nih.gov/36094001/.
https://pubmed.ncbi.nlm.nih.gov/28531358/. https://pubmed.ncbi.nlm.nih.gov/32314650/.
https://pubmed.ncbi.nlm.nih.gov/22891006/.
910. Articles: https://pubmed.ncbi.nlm.nih.gov/36094001/.
https://pubmed.ncbi.nlm.nih.gov/28531358/. https://pubmed.ncbi.nlm.nih.gov/32314650/.
https://pubmed.ncbi.nlm.nih.gov/22891006/.
911. Articles: https://pubmed.ncbi.nlm.nih.gov/20301505/.
https://pubmed.ncbi.nlm.nih.gov/29101669/. https://pubmed.ncbi.nlm.nih.gov/32316673/.
https://pubmed.ncbi.nlm.nih.gov/26873308/. https://pubmed.ncbi.nlm.nih.gov/36708456/.
912. Articles: https://pubmed.ncbi.nlm.nih.gov/1911337/.
https://www.sciencedirect.com/topics/medicine-and-dentistry/pityriasis-rubra-pilaris.
913. Articles: https://pubmed.ncbi.nlm.nih.gov/31526611/.
https://pubmed.ncbi.nlm.nih.gov/31340689/. https://pubmed.ncbi.nlm.nih.gov/29057843/.

914. Articles: https://pubmed.ncbi.nlm.nih.gov/32443760/.
https://pubmed.ncbi.nlm.nih.gov/30322097/. https://pubmed.ncbi.nlm.nih.gov/26765344/.
https://pubmed.ncbi.nlm.nih.gov/33232955/. https://pubmed.ncbi.nlm.nih.gov/30089075/.
915. Articles: https://www.sciencedaily.com/releases/2022/10/221026102935.htm.
https://pubmed.ncbi.nlm.nih.gov/36279545/. https://pubmed.ncbi.nlm.nih.gov/38086258/.
916. Articles: https://pubmed.ncbi.nlm.nih.gov/27479626/.
https://pubmed.ncbi.nlm.nih.gov/36819682/. https://pubmed.ncbi.nlm.nih.gov/22010771/.
https://pubmed.ncbi.nlm.nih.gov/26724745/. https://pubmed.ncbi.nlm.nih.gov/39071517/.
https://pubmed.ncbi.nlm.nih.gov/38931266/.
917. Vitamin D has been show to ease the symptoms of PMS. Altshul and Hops, p. 290. Articles:
https://pubmed.ncbi.nlm.nih.gov/29447494/. https://pubmed.ncbi.nlm.nih.gov/30918875/.
https://pubmed.ncbi.nlm.nih.gov/35065636/. https://pubmed.ncbi.nlm.nih.gov/38220382/.
918. Articles: https://pubmed.ncbi.nlm.nih.gov/38345088/.
https://pubmed.ncbi.nlm.nih.gov/34323091/. https://pubmed.ncbi.nlm.nih.gov/21966215/.
https://pubmed.ncbi.nlm.nih.gov/29241179/. https://pubmed.ncbi.nlm.nih.gov/30101993/.
https://pubmed.ncbi.nlm.nih.gov/32654618/.
919. Articles: https://pubmed.ncbi.nlm.nih.gov/33232955/.
https://pubmed.ncbi.nlm.nih.gov/35565867/. https://pubmed.ncbi.nlm.nih.gov/36296914/.
https://pubmed.ncbi.nlm.nih.gov/31348529/.
920. Articles: https://pubmed.ncbi.nlm.nih.gov/7041638/.
https://pubmed.ncbi.nlm.nih.gov/32533118/. https://pubmed.ncbi.nlm.nih.gov/10435676/.
https://pubmed.ncbi.nlm.nih.gov/7041638/. https://pubmed.ncbi.nlm.nih.gov/5618332/.
921. Articles: https://www.ncbi.nlm.nih.gov/pmc/articles/PMC5207540/.
https://www.aware.app/magazine/the-science-of-vitamin-d-how-it-improves-energy-mood#:~:text=
Research%20suggests%20vitamin%20D%20supports,leads%20to%20improved%20energy%20levels.
https://ro.co/supplements/does-vitamin-d-give-you-energy/.
922. Articles: https://pn.bmj.com/content/21/5/376.
https://www.ncbi.nlm.nih.gov/pmc/articles/PMC8530200/.
https://pspawareness.com/blogs/psp-q-a/nutrition-and-psp.
923. Related article: https://pubmed.ncbi.nlm.nih.gov/9711982/.
924. Because it can suppress the growth of cancer cells, vitamin D has been found to be successful in both
preventing and treating a myriad of cancers. *Food and Nutrition*, p. 30; see also Dowd and Stafford, pp.
171-173; Zaidi, pp. 106-114. Articles: https://pubmed.ncbi.nlm.nih.gov/29667615/.
https://pubmed.ncbi.nlm.nih.gov/26827958/. https://pubmed.ncbi.nlm.nih.gov/29765146/.
https://pubmed.ncbi.nlm.nih.gov/35761063/. https://pubmed.ncbi.nlm.nih.gov/14580762/.
925. Articles: https://pubmed.ncbi.nlm.nih.gov/23930605/.
https://academic.oup.com/jcem/article/97/7/2315/2834130.
https://lcm.amegroups.org/article/view/8139/html#:~:text=Low%20(25%2DOH)%20vitamin,with
%20serum%20PSA%20(34).
https://journals.lww.com/oncology-times/fulltext/2015/04250/evidence_that_vitamin_d_can_slow_
or_reverse.20.aspx.
926. Articles: https://pubmed.ncbi.nlm.nih.gov/22544696/.
https://pubmed.ncbi.nlm.nih.gov/25609737/. https://pubmed.ncbi.nlm.nih.gov/23929770/.
https://pubmed.ncbi.nlm.nih.gov/33026128/.
927. Related articles: https://pubmed.ncbi.nlm.nih.gov/12100455/.
https://pubmed.ncbi.nlm.nih.gov/32347013/.
928. Related articles: https://pubmed.ncbi.nlm.nih.gov/16357816/.
https://pubmed.ncbi.nlm.nih.gov/20181799/.
929. Articles: https://pubmed.ncbi.nlm.nih.gov/36246903/.
https://pubmed.ncbi.nlm.nih.gov/37500374/. https://pubmed.ncbi.nlm.nih.gov/33130042/.
https://pubmed.ncbi.nlm.nih.gov/183579/. https://pubmed.ncbi.nlm.nih.gov/21274319/.
https://pubmed.ncbi.nlm.nih.gov/2724638/.
930. Vitamin D has been used successfully to treat psoriasis. *Food and Nutrition*, p. 30; Altshul and Hops.
p. 312. Articles: https://pubmed.ncbi.nlm.nih.gov/35955731/.
https://pubmed.ncbi.nlm.nih.gov/37571324/. https://pubmed.ncbi.nlm.nih.gov/33419149/.
https://pubmed.ncbi.nlm.nih.gov/25601579/.
931. Articles: https://pubmed.ncbi.nlm.nih.gov/19818218/.
https://pubmed.ncbi.nlm.nih.gov/38009028/. https://pubmed.ncbi.nlm.nih.gov/36108165/.
932. Articles: https://pubmed.ncbi.nlm.nih.gov/37062151/.
https://pubmed.ncbi.nlm.nih.gov/36214524/. https://pubmed.ncbi.nlm.nih.gov/36398080/.

933. Articles: https://pn.bmj.com/content/21/5/376.
https://www.ncbi.nlm.nih.gov/pmc/articles/PMC8530200/.
https://pspawareness.com/blogs/psp-q-a/nutrition-and-psp.
934. Articles: https://www.ncbi.nlm.nih.gov/pmc/articles/PMC4511535/.
https://pubmed.ncbi.nlm.nih.gov/26203431/.
935. Articles: https://www.ncbi.nlm.nih.gov/pmc/articles/PMC8584834/.
https://www.promises.com/addiction-blog/does-vitamin-d-play-a-role-in-psychiatry/.
https://www.webmd.com/vitamins-and-supplements/what-to-know-about-vitamin-d-and-mental-healt
h. https://www.ncbi.nlm.nih.gov/pmc/articles/PMC6525761/.
https://www.ncbi.nlm.nih.gov/pmc/articles/PMC6525761/.
https://bmcpsychiatry.biomedcentral.com/articles/10.1186/1471-244X-12-38.
https://www.sciencedirect.com/science/article/abs/pii/S0278584619302258.
https://jamanetwork.com/journals/jamanetworkopen/fullarticle/2787456.
https://www.vitamind-journal.it/en/wp-content/uploads/2019/04/03_Fagiolini_1_19_EN-2.pdf.
936. Article: https://pubmed.ncbi.nlm.nih.gov/28202197/.
937. Related articles:
https://www.webmd.com/vitamins-and-supplements/what-to-know-about-vitamin-d-and-mental-healt
h. https://www.vitamind-journal.it/en/wp-content/uploads/2019/04/03_Fagiolini_1_19_EN-2.pdf.
https://psychcentral.com/blog/does-vitamin-d-deficiency-impact-mental-health.
https://bmcpsychiatry.biomedcentral.com/articles/10.1186/1471-244X-12-38.
938. Articles: https://pubmed.ncbi.nlm.nih.gov/27245208/.
https://pubmed.ncbi.nlm.nih.gov/26005122/.
939. Articles: https://pubmed.ncbi.nlm.nih.gov/34999745/.
https://pubmed.ncbi.nlm.nih.gov/31093951/. https://pubmed.ncbi.nlm.nih.gov/25713056/.
https://pubmed.ncbi.nlm.nih.gov/33049684/. https://pubmed.ncbi.nlm.nih.gov/35156551/.
https://pubmed.ncbi.nlm.nih.gov/35311615/.
940. Articles: https://pubmed.ncbi.nlm.nih.gov/33049684/.
https://pubmed.ncbi.nlm.nih.gov/23906618/. https://pubmed.ncbi.nlm.nih.gov/33838984/.
https://pubmed.ncbi.nlm.nih.gov/37850995/. https://pubmed.ncbi.nlm.nih.gov/31262684/.
https://pubmed.ncbi.nlm.nih.gov/31187033/. https://pubmed.ncbi.nlm.nih.gov/30154029/.
https://pubmed.ncbi.nlm.nih.gov/30142216/.
941. Articles: https://pubmed.ncbi.nlm.nih.gov/31518608/.
https://pubmed.ncbi.nlm.nih.gov/37685345/.
https://www.sciencedirect.com/science/article/abs/pii/S0278584619305184#:~:text=PTSD%20is
%20associated%20with%20reduced,adjusting%20for%20vitamin%20D%20levels.
https://pubmed.ncbi.nlm.nih.gov/24604440/.
https://www.drjonslaughter.com/post/the-benefits-of-vitamin-d-in-depression-and-ptsd.
https://www.mdpi.com/2075-4418/13/17/2807.
942. Articles: https://pubmed.ncbi.nlm.nih.gov/36562273/.
https://pubmed.ncbi.nlm.nih.gov/35383823/. https://pubmed.ncbi.nlm.nih.gov/37353234/.
https://pubmed.ncbi.nlm.nih.gov/27925404/.
943. Articles: https://pubmed.ncbi.nlm.nih.gov/37575807/.
https://pubmed.ncbi.nlm.nih.gov/31974323/. https://pubmed.ncbi.nlm.nih.gov/31974323/.
944. Articles: https://pubmed.ncbi.nlm.nih.gov/31934161/.
https://pubmed.ncbi.nlm.nih.gov/35906886/. https://pubmed.ncbi.nlm.nih.gov/37612740/.
https://pubmed.ncbi.nlm.nih.gov/34400742/. https://pubmed.ncbi.nlm.nih.gov/31775746/.
945. Articles: https://pubmed.ncbi.nlm.nih.gov/38008680/.
https://pubmed.ncbi.nlm.nih.gov/29057843/. https://pubmed.ncbi.nlm.nih.gov/37405341/.
https://pubmed.ncbi.nlm.nih.gov/31864342/. https://pubmed.ncbi.nlm.nih.gov/37808898/.
946. Related articles: https://pubmed.ncbi.nlm.nih.gov/37919813/.
https://pubmed.ncbi.nlm.nih.gov/25130505/. https://pubmed.ncbi.nlm.nih.gov/8305916/.
https://pubmed.ncbi.nlm.nih.gov/29417593/.
947. Article: https://pubmed.ncbi.nlm.nih.gov/37501941/.
948. Related article: https://pubmed.ncbi.nlm.nih.gov/5773282/.
949. Article: https://pubmed.ncbi.nlm.nih.gov/30258025/.
950. Articles:
https://www.researchgate.net/publication/339913302_Paediatric_gastric_trichobezoar_the_Rapunzel
_syndrome_A_report_of_two_cases.
https://www.anncaserep.com/open-access/association-of-pediatric-rapunzel-syndrome-with-proteinlos
ing-enteropathybr-nbsp-6030.pdf.

https://www.degruyter.com/document/doi/10.1515/med-2020-0243/html?lang=en.
https://www.emjreviews.com/dermatology/article/trichotillomania-with-giant-gastric-trichobezoar-in
-a-female-child-a-case-report/.
951. Articles: https://pubmed.ncbi.nlm.nih.gov/22580932/.
https://pubmed.ncbi.nlm.nih.gov/35488070/. https://pubmed.ncbi.nlm.nih.gov/30050814/.
https://pubmed.ncbi.nlm.nih.gov/34132891/. https://pubmed.ncbi.nlm.nih.gov/23918994/.
952. Articles: https://pubmed.ncbi.nlm.nih.gov/36793500/.
https://pubmed.ncbi.nlm.nih.gov/37739725/. https://pubmed.ncbi.nlm.nih.gov/26751969/.
https://pubmed.ncbi.nlm.nih.gov/23323190/. https://pubmed.ncbi.nlm.nih.gov/37434995/.
953. Related articles: https://pubmed.ncbi.nlm.nih.gov/25616861/.
954. Related articles: https://www.ncbi.nlm.nih.gov/pmc/articles/PMC2853984/.
https://ajronline.org/doi/full/10.2214/AJR.09.3130.
https://onlinelibrary.wiley.com/doi/pdf/10.1002/jcsm.12364.
955. Articles: https://pubmed.ncbi.nlm.nih.gov/32679784/.
https://pubmed.ncbi.nlm.nih.gov/30614127/. https://pubmed.ncbi.nlm.nih.gov/26521023/.
956. Articles: https://pubmed.ncbi.nlm.nih.gov/3755603/.
https://pubmed.ncbi.nlm.nih.gov/9090766/. Related article:
https://pubmed.ncbi.nlm.nih.gov/6287592/.
957. Articles: https://pubmed.ncbi.nlm.nih.gov/28346348/.
https://pubmed.ncbi.nlm.nih.gov/17197169/. https://pubmed.ncbi.nlm.nih.gov/12109997/.
https://pubmed.ncbi.nlm.nih.gov/12401838/.
958. Articles: https://pubmed.ncbi.nlm.nih.gov/33774081/.
https://pubmed.ncbi.nlm.nih.gov/36173905/. https://pubmed.ncbi.nlm.nih.gov/33190187/.
https://pubmed.ncbi.nlm.nih.gov/3037668/. https://pubmed.ncbi.nlm.nih.gov/15577104/.
https://pubmed.ncbi.nlm.nih.gov/1599820/.
959. Articles: https://pubmed.ncbi.nlm.nih.gov/26521023/.
https://pubmed.ncbi.nlm.nih.gov/37571367/. https://pubmed.ncbi.nlm.nih.gov/27009076/.
960. Articles: https://pubmed.ncbi.nlm.nih.gov/37034443/.
https://pubmed.ncbi.nlm.nih.gov/36187108/. https://pubmed.ncbi.nlm.nih.gov/36377836/.
https://pubmed.ncbi.nlm.nih.gov/34867766/. https://pubmed.ncbi.nlm.nih.gov/32078093/.
https://pubmed.ncbi.nlm.nih.gov/30430372/.
961. Articles: https://pubmed.ncbi.nlm.nih.gov/37005543/.
https://pubmed.ncbi.nlm.nih.gov/12324873/. https://pubmed.ncbi.nlm.nih.gov/2833210/.
https://pubmed.ncbi.nlm.nih.gov/34444670/. https://pubmed.ncbi.nlm.nih.gov/14507860/.
https://pubmed.ncbi.nlm.nih.gov/1634333/.
962. Articles: https://pubmed.ncbi.nlm.nih.gov/37569392/.
https://pubmed.ncbi.nlm.nih.gov/35457041/. https://pubmed.ncbi.nlm.nih.gov/37085359/.
https://pubmed.ncbi.nlm.nih.gov/36349170/. https://pubmed.ncbi.nlm.nih.gov/32308951/.
https://pubmed.ncbi.nlm.nih.gov/33760363/. https://pubmed.ncbi.nlm.nih.gov/28457295/.
https://pubmed.ncbi.nlm.nih.gov/35673423/.
963. Articles: https://pubmed.ncbi.nlm.nih.gov/35710090/.
https://pubmed.ncbi.nlm.nih.gov/22550417/. https://pubmed.ncbi.nlm.nih.gov/8646514/.
https://pubmed.ncbi.nlm.nih.gov/2009222/.
964. Articles: https://pubmed.ncbi.nlm.nih.gov/31286174/.
https://pubmed.ncbi.nlm.nih.gov/34827621/. https://pubmed.ncbi.nlm.nih.gov/26481434/. See
also Holick, pp. 107-109.
965. Articles: https://pubmed.ncbi.nlm.nih.gov/36866055/.
https://pubmed.ncbi.nlm.nih.gov/36137920/. https://pubmed.ncbi.nlm.nih.gov/11176917/.
966. Articles: https://pubmed.ncbi.nlm.nih.gov/24748637/.
https://pubmed.ncbi.nlm.nih.gov/34969941/. https://pubmed.ncbi.nlm.nih.gov/33232959/.
967. Articles: https://pubmed.ncbi.nlm.nih.gov/33476988/.
https://www.ijord.com/index.php/ijord/article/view/1103.
https://www.producer.com/livestock/vitamins-solve-ringworm-problem/#:~:text=Healthy%20skin
%20is%20a%20great,which%20helps%20kill%20this%20organism. Related:
https://www.healthline.com/health/fungal-infection/which-vitamin-deficiency-causes-fungal-infection.
968. Vitamin D may help treat RMSF by building up the immune system. L.S. Article:
https://www.jillcarnahan.com/2021/05/04/protect-yourself-from-rocky-mountain-spotted-fever/.
969. Vitamin D may help treat RMSF by building up the immune system. L.S. Article:
https://www.jillcarnahan.com/2021/05/04/protect-yourself-from-rocky-mountain-spotted-fever/.

970. Articles: https://pubmed.ncbi.nlm.nih.gov/37686836/.
https://pubmed.ncbi.nlm.nih.gov/23713748/. https://pubmed.ncbi.nlm.nih.gov/36636389/.
https://pubmed.ncbi.nlm.nih.gov/29606809/. https://pubmed.ncbi.nlm.nih.gov/30246390/.
https://pubmed.ncbi.nlm.nih.gov/15187348/.
971. Articles: https://pubmed.ncbi.nlm.nih.gov/27366101/.
https://pubmed.ncbi.nlm.nih.gov/30850081/. https://pubmed.ncbi.nlm.nih.gov/37449678/.
972. Articles: https://pubmed.ncbi.nlm.nih.gov/28796426/.
https://pubmed.ncbi.nlm.nih.gov/15702407/. https://pubmed.ncbi.nlm.nih.gov/33838771/.
https://pubmed.ncbi.nlm.nih.gov/29355488/.
973. Article: https://pubmed.ncbi.nlm.nih.gov/36245733/.
974. Articles: https://pubmed.ncbi.nlm.nih.gov/38931257/.
https://pubmed.ncbi.nlm.nih.gov/9539254/.
https://healthmatch.io/seasonal-affective-disorder/vitamin-d-for-seasonal-depression.
https://pubmed.ncbi.nlm.nih.gov/25270233/.
https://www.ssmhealth.com/newsroom/blogs/ssm-health-matters/march-2022/low-levels-of-vitamin
-d-can-increase-your-risk-of.
https://www.healthline.com/health/depression/vitamins-for-seasonal-depression. See also Holick, pp.
122-123.
975. Articles: https://www.ncbi.nlm.nih.gov/pmc/articles/PMC4511535/. See also:
https://pubmed.ncbi.nlm.nih.gov/26724745/. https://pubmed.ncbi.nlm.nih.gov/32215634/.
976. Articles: https://pubmed.ncbi.nlm.nih.gov/34576700/.
https://pubmed.ncbi.nlm.nih.gov/33559391/. https://pubmed.ncbi.nlm.nih.gov/34680413/.
https://pubmed.ncbi.nlm.nih.gov/36678175/.
977. Articles: https://pubmed.ncbi.nlm.nih.gov/33659946/.
https://pubmed.ncbi.nlm.nih.gov/28323225/. https://pubmed.ncbi.nlm.nih.gov/20671517/.
https://pubmed.ncbi.nlm.nih.gov/20665397/.
978. Articles: https://pubmed.ncbi.nlm.nih.gov/31766576/.
https://pubmed.ncbi.nlm.nih.gov/35406137/. https://pubmed.ncbi.nlm.nih.gov/33086536/.
https://pubmed.ncbi.nlm.nih.gov/32219739/.
979. Related article: https://www.ncbi.nlm.nih.gov/pmc/articles/PMC5051481/.
980. Articles: https://pubmed.ncbi.nlm.nih.gov/36819669/.
https://pubmed.ncbi.nlm.nih.gov/34864844/. https://pubmed.ncbi.nlm.nih.gov/34369338/.
981. Articles: https://pubmed.ncbi.nlm.nih.gov/21992906/.
https://pubmed.ncbi.nlm.nih.gov/22612551/.
982. Article: https://www.ncbi.nlm.nih.gov/pmc/articles/PMC7710713/. Related article:
https://pubmed.ncbi.nlm.nih.gov/20336615/.
https://dergipark.org.tr/tr/download/article-file/466118.
983. Article: https://pubmed.ncbi.nlm.nih.gov/17357880/.
984. Articles: https://pubmed.ncbi.nlm.nih.gov/25713056/.
https://pubmed.ncbi.nlm.nih.gov/33500553/. https://pubmed.ncbi.nlm.nih.gov/32912355/.
https://pubmed.ncbi.nlm.nih.gov/26767392/. https://pubmed.ncbi.nlm.nih.gov/28396640/.
985. Related articles: https://www.ncbi.nlm.nih.gov/pmc/articles/PMC8505257/.
https://www.ncbi.nlm.nih.gov/pmc/articles/PMC4257987/.
https://www.psychiatrictimes.com/view/study-finds-that-probiotics-vitamin-d-may-enhance-cognitive-
function-in-schizophrenia. https://jamanetwork.com/journals/jamanetworkopen/fullarticle/2787456.
986. Articles:
https://prochiromt.com/best-vitamins-for-sciatic-nerve-pain/#:~:text=Studies%20suggest%20that%2
0increasing%20vitamin,discomfort%20associated%20with%20sciatic%20pain.
https://pubmed.ncbi.nlm.nih.gov/34378677/.
https://www.spine-health.com/blog/5-tips-relieve-sciatica-pain.
987. Articles: https://pubmed.ncbi.nlm.nih.gov/36813139/.
https://pubmed.ncbi.nlm.nih.gov/32563782/. https://pubmed.ncbi.nlm.nih.gov/36235561/.
988. Articles: https://pubmed.ncbi.nlm.nih.gov/37644501/.
https://pubmed.ncbi.nlm.nih.gov/37886647/. https://pubmed.ncbi.nlm.nih.gov/36764946/.
https://pubmed.ncbi.nlm.nih.gov/33683641/. https://pubmed.ncbi.nlm.nih.gov/27089048/.
989. Articles: https://pubmed.ncbi.nlm.nih.gov/38931257/.
https://pubmed.ncbi.nlm.nih.gov/9539254/.
https://healthmatch.io/seasonal-affective-disorder/vitamin-d-for-seasonal-depression.
https://pubmed.ncbi.nlm.nih.gov/25270233/.
https://www.ssmhealth.com/newsroom/blogs/ssm-health-matters/march-2022/low-levels-of-vitamin

-d-can-increase-your-risk-of.
https://www.healthline.com/health/depression/vitamins-for-seasonal-depression. See also Holick, pp. 122-123.
990. Articles: https://pubmed.ncbi.nlm.nih.gov/37607492/.
https://pubmed.ncbi.nlm.nih.gov/24667068/. https://pubmed.ncbi.nlm.nih.gov/30225226/.
991. Related articles:
https://thedawnrehab.com/blog/12-supplements-that-benefit-recovery-from-addiction/.
https://www.paracelsus-recovery.com/blog/vitamin-d-and-addiction/.
992. Articles: https://pubmed.ncbi.nlm.nih.gov/23859137/.
https://dpcj.org/index.php/dpc/article/view/3245.
https://www.semanticscholar.org/paper/The-roles-of-vitamin-D-in-seborrhoeic-keratosis%3A-L%C6
%B0%C6%A1ng-Nguy%E1%BB%85n/cfbb22d84dd66b214452f851331df2eb18e741f7.
993. Related articles: https://pubmed.ncbi.nlm.nih.gov/34095485/.
https://pubmed.ncbi.nlm.nih.gov/22512666/. https://pubmed.ncbi.nlm.nih.gov/33318252/.
994. Article: https://journals.plos.org/plosone/article?id=10.1371/journal.pone.0279166.
995. Articles: https://pubmed.ncbi.nlm.nih.gov/23135697/.
https://www.ncbi.nlm.nih.gov/pmc/articles/PMC4427945/.
https://www.ncbi.nlm.nih.gov/pmc/articles/PMC7270292/.
996. Articles: https://pubmed.ncbi.nlm.nih.gov/37498186/.
https://pubmed.ncbi.nlm.nih.gov/35779352/. https://pubmed.ncbi.nlm.nih.gov/33777323/.
https://pubmed.ncbi.nlm.nih.gov/38529449/.
997. Articles: https://pubmed.ncbi.nlm.nih.gov/36769240/.
https://pubmed.ncbi.nlm.nih.gov/31495735/. https://pubmed.ncbi.nlm.nih.gov/30021102/.
https://pubmed.ncbi.nlm.nih.gov/37892385/.
998. Articles: https://pubmed.ncbi.nlm.nih.gov/23889483/.
https://pubmed.ncbi.nlm.nih.gov/30006615/. https://pubmed.ncbi.nlm.nih.gov/30470461/.
https://pubmed.ncbi.nlm.nih.gov/28335672/.
999. Articles: https://pubmed.ncbi.nlm.nih.gov/36819669/.
https://pubmed.ncbi.nlm.nih.gov/34864844/. https://pubmed.ncbi.nlm.nih.gov/34369338/.
1000. Related articles: https://www.ncbi.nlm.nih.gov/pmc/articles/PMC6521317/.
https://www.nature.com/articles/s41380-021-01025-0.
https://mosaicdx.com/resource/the-effect-of-vitamin-d-on-psychosis-and-schizophrenia/.
https://www.ncbi.nlm.nih.gov/pmc/articles/PMC6693492/.
1001. Articles: https://pubmed.ncbi.nlm.nih.gov/33511224/.
https://pubmed.ncbi.nlm.nih.gov/35940884/. https://pubmed.ncbi.nlm.nih.gov/31594899/.
1002. Articles: https://pubmed.ncbi.nlm.nih.gov/31941599/.
https://pubmed.ncbi.nlm.nih.gov/27589260/.
1003. Related articles: https://pubmed.ncbi.nlm.nih.gov/36694870/.
https://pubmed.ncbi.nlm.nih.gov/37116013/. https://pubmed.ncbi.nlm.nih.gov/20954138/.
1004. Related articles: https://pubmed.ncbi.nlm.nih.gov/35458189/.
https://pubmed.ncbi.nlm.nih.gov/34104581/. https://pubmed.ncbi.nlm.nih.gov/32883903/.
https://pubmed.ncbi.nlm.nih.gov/34462708/.
1005. Articles: https://www.ncbi.nlm.nih.gov/pmc/articles/PMC4922356/.
https://www.tandfonline.com/doi/full/10.1080/16089677.2023.2178155.
https://pubmed.ncbi.nlm.nih.gov/34522473/. https://pubmed.ncbi.nlm.nih.gov/22218780/.
https://pubmed.ncbi.nlm.nih.gov/36188735/.
1006. Articles: https://pubmed.ncbi.nlm.nih.gov/34267848/.
https://pubmed.ncbi.nlm.nih.gov/30520760/.
1007. Articles: https://pubmed.ncbi.nlm.nih.gov/20301551/.
https://pubmed.ncbi.nlm.nih.gov/28105733/. https://pubmed.ncbi.nlm.nih.gov/32462740/.
https://pubmed.ncbi.nlm.nih.gov/28259214/.
1008. Related articles: https://pubmed.ncbi.nlm.nih.gov/2379840/.
https://pubmed.ncbi.nlm.nih.gov/37404402/.
1009. Articles: https://pubmed.ncbi.nlm.nih.gov/9212183/.
https://pubmed.ncbi.nlm.nih.gov/3474327/.
1010. Articles: https://pubmed.ncbi.nlm.nih.gov/12710640/.
https://pubmed.ncbi.nlm.nih.gov/23600989/. https://pubmed.ncbi.nlm.nih.gov/6966389/.
https://pubmed.ncbi.nlm.nih.gov/25019937/. https://pubmed.ncbi.nlm.nih.gov/10434505/.
https://pubmed.ncbi.nlm.nih.gov/10459231/.

1011. Articles: https://pubmed.ncbi.nlm.nih.gov/27466850/.
https://pubmed.ncbi.nlm.nih.gov/34198970/. https://pubmed.ncbi.nlm.nih.gov/22193052/.
https://pubmed.ncbi.nlm.nih.gov/37109265/. https://pubmed.ncbi.nlm.nih.gov/26623567/.
https://pubmed.ncbi.nlm.nih.gov/33170652/.

1012. Articles: https://pubmed.ncbi.nlm.nih.gov/37189455/.
https://pubmed.ncbi.nlm.nih.gov/37189174/. https://pubmed.ncbi.nlm.nih.gov/28411165/.
https://pubmed.ncbi.nlm.nih.gov/32172354/. https://pubmed.ncbi.nlm.nih.gov/36771203/.
https://pubmed.ncbi.nlm.nih.gov/35611106/. https://pubmed.ncbi.nlm.nih.gov/29207757/.

1013. Articles: https://pubmed.ncbi.nlm.nih.gov/28994020/.
https://pubmed.ncbi.nlm.nih.gov/29249122/. https://pubmed.ncbi.nlm.nih.gov/31892603/.
https://pubmed.ncbi.nlm.nih.gov/21371954/. https://pubmed.ncbi.nlm.nih.gov/32918212/.

1014. Articles: https://pubmed.ncbi.nlm.nih.gov/34638299/.
https://pubmed.ncbi.nlm.nih.gov/38138233/. https://pubmed.ncbi.nlm.nih.gov/34631325/.
https://pubmed.ncbi.nlm.nih.gov/37237973/. https://pubmed.ncbi.nlm.nih.gov/25087185/.
https://pubmed.ncbi.nlm.nih.gov/18267352/. https://pubmed.ncbi.nlm.nih.gov/33255834/.

1015. Articles: https://pubmed.ncbi.nlm.nih.gov/28994020/.
https://pubmed.ncbi.nlm.nih.gov/32360756/. https://pubmed.ncbi.nlm.nih.gov/21034990/.
https://pubmed.ncbi.nlm.nih.gov/29306952/. https://pubmed.ncbi.nlm.nih.gov/30857638/.
https://pubmed.ncbi.nlm.nih.gov/34785011/.

1016. Articles: https://pubmed.ncbi.nlm.nih.gov/21133662/.
https://pubmed.ncbi.nlm.nih.gov/31302984/. https://pubmed.ncbi.nlm.nih.gov/32918212/.

1017. Related articles: https://pubmed.ncbi.nlm.nih.gov/28477263/.
https://pubmed.ncbi.nlm.nih.gov/35895040/.

1018. Article:
https://www.kairoswellnesscollective.com/blog/best-supplements-for-skin-picking-disorder.

1019. Since vitamin D deficiency is related to insulin resistance and diabetes, and because skin tags are associated with diabetes, it will not be surprising if skin tags also turn out to be connected to a vitamin D deficiency. See, for example, the following articles: https://pubmed.ncbi.nlm.nih.gov/15186199/.
https://www.ncbi.nlm.nih.gov/pmc/articles/PMC2947742/.

1020. Articles: https://www.ncbi.nlm.nih.gov/pmc/articles/PMC6493208/. Related article:
https://sunsaferx.com/blogs/health-wellness/erythema-treatment-prevention.

1021. Vitamin D deficiency has been linked to autoimmune-inflammatory diseases like lupus. Because lupus patients must avoid exposure to the sun, adequate vitamin D from other sources is imperative for good health. Weiss, p. 221. Articles: https://pubmed.ncbi.nlm.nih.gov/35648165/.
https://pubmed.ncbi.nlm.nih.gov/37189455/. https://pubmed.ncbi.nlm.nih.gov/29108830/.

1022. Articles: https://pubmed.ncbi.nlm.nih.gov/35163353/.
https://pubmed.ncbi.nlm.nih.gov/37704922/. https://pubmed.ncbi.nlm.nih.gov/38414320/.
https://pubmed.ncbi.nlm.nih.gov/37322405/. https://pubmed.ncbi.nlm.nih.gov/30186518/.

1023. Articles: https://pubmed.ncbi.nlm.nih.gov/32156230/.
https://pubmed.ncbi.nlm.nih.gov/32987320/. https://pubmed.ncbi.nlm.nih.gov/35268051/.
https://pubmed.ncbi.nlm.nih.gov/35578558/. https://pubmed.ncbi.nlm.nih.gov/32672533/.

1024. The proper amount of vitamin D will provide most people with a night of rich, enjoyable, and fulfilling sleep. In addition, one usually sleeps longer and deeper, dream quality improves, and nightmares disappear. I can personally testify to this. L.S. Articles:
https://www.ncbi.nlm.nih.gov/pmc/articles/PMC4511535/.
https://pubmed.ncbi.nlm.nih.gov/35578558/.

1025. Articles:
https://go.gale.com/ps/i.do?id=GALE%7CA600665928&sid=googleScholar&v=2.1&it=r&linkaccess=abs&issn=21492247&p=AONE&sw=w&userGroupName=anon%7E910983e1&aty=open-web-entry#:~:text=Children%20with%20sleep%20terror%20with,among%20children%20with%20sleep%20terror.
https://www.researchgate.net/publication/334054145_Vitamin_D_Levels_in_Children_with_Sleep_Terror_Analytical_Cross-Sectional_Study.
https://omegaquant.com/the-role-of-vitamins-in-promoting-restful-sleep/.
https://search.trdizin.gov.tr/tr/yayin/detay/320178/vitamin-d-levels-in-children-with-sleep-terror-analytical-cross-sectional-study.
https://www.drugs.com/comments/cholecalciferol/for-vitamin-d-deficiency.html?page=2.
https://www.healthcentral.com/condition/night-terrors.

1026. Related article: https://www.ncbi.nlm.nih.gov/pmc/articles/PMC6213953/.

1027. Article: https://pubmed.ncbi.nlm.nih.gov/20736407/.
https://www.scielo.org.za/scielo.php?script=sci_arttext&pid=S1681-150X2011000200007.
1028. Articles: https://www.ncbi.nlm.nih.gov/pmc/articles/PMC3315864/.
https://www.sciencedirect.com/science/article/abs/pii/S155637071100157X.
https://www.cambridge.org/core/journals/journal-of-laryngology-and-otology/article/abs/vitamin-d-and-smell-impairment-a-systematic-literature-review/AEB7BBD23006DF87042802BA73250D41.
1029. Articles: https://pubmed.ncbi.nlm.nih.gov/28796426/.
https://pubmed.ncbi.nlm.nih.gov/15702407/. https://pubmed.ncbi.nlm.nih.gov/33838771/.
https://pubmed.ncbi.nlm.nih.gov/29355488/.
1030. Articles: https://pubmed.ncbi.nlm.nih.gov/2204648/.
https://pubmed.ncbi.nlm.nih.gov/28079559/. https://pubmed.ncbi.nlm.nih.gov/2204648/.
https://pubmed.ncbi.nlm.nih.gov/27035899/. https://pubmed.ncbi.nlm.nih.gov/23888288/.
1031. Article: https://pubmed.ncbi.nlm.nih.gov/35156551/.
1032. Articles: https://pubmed.ncbi.nlm.nih.gov/25667508/.
https://pubmed.ncbi.nlm.nih.gov/8646514/.
1033. Article: https://pubmed.ncbi.nlm.nih.gov/30416297/.
1034. Related articles: https://pubmed.ncbi.nlm.nih.gov/37900412/.
https://pubmed.ncbi.nlm.nih.gov/33292313/. https://pubmed.ncbi.nlm.nih.gov/26521023/.
1035. Articles: https://www.ncbi.nlm.nih.gov/pmc/articles/PMC4021247/.
https://www.e-aair.org/pdf/10.4168/aair.2014.6.3.267.
https://www.ncbi.nlm.nih.gov/pmc/articles/PMC9771342/.
https://pubmed.ncbi.nlm.nih.gov/36550807/. Video:
https://www.youtube.com/watch?v=zCmW5bLcE9s.
1036. Articles: https://pubmed.ncbi.nlm.nih.gov/31496497/.
https://www.theglenfieldsurgery.co.uk/website/C82056/files/VITAMIN%20D%20DEFICIENCY.pdf
. https://www.medicinenet.com/symptoms_and_causes_of_vitamin_d_deficiency/article.htm.
1037. Articles: https://pubmed.ncbi.nlm.nih.gov/22083799/.
https://pubmed.ncbi.nlm.nih.gov/24948020/.
1038. Articles: https://pubmed.ncbi.nlm.nih.gov/?term=vitamin+d+Spinal+Cord+Disease.
https://pubmed.ncbi.nlm.nih.gov/34921084/. https://pubmed.ncbi.nlm.nih.gov/29424660/.
https://pubmed.ncbi.nlm.nih.gov/36581746/. https://pubmed.ncbi.nlm.nih.gov/36843972/.
1039. Related articles: https://pubmed.ncbi.nlm.nih.gov/20301551/.
https://pubmed.ncbi.nlm.nih.gov/36893148/. https://pubmed.ncbi.nlm.nih.gov/1775519/.
1040. Articles: https://pubmed.ncbi.nlm.nih.gov/25860535/.
https://pubmed.ncbi.nlm.nih.gov/37407993/. https://pubmed.ncbi.nlm.nih.gov/34289005/.
1041. Articles: https://pubmed.ncbi.nlm.nih.gov/19835345/.
https://pubmed.ncbi.nlm.nih.gov/20051755/. https://pubmed.ncbi.nlm.nih.gov/25202161/.
1042. Articles: https://pubmed.ncbi.nlm.nih.gov/37198534/.
https://pubmed.ncbi.nlm.nih.gov/28306725/. https://pubmed.ncbi.nlm.nih.gov/27308854/.
1043. Articles: https://pubmed.ncbi.nlm.nih.gov/12827405/.
https://pubmed.ncbi.nlm.nih.gov/32277367/.
1044. Articles: https://pubmed.ncbi.nlm.nih.gov/34766885/.
https://pubmed.ncbi.nlm.nih.gov/31757059/. Related article:
https://pubmed.ncbi.nlm.nih.gov/31757059/.
1045. Articles: https://pubmed.ncbi.nlm.nih.gov/29403195/.
https://pubmed.ncbi.nlm.nih.gov/37334809/. https://pubmed.ncbi.nlm.nih.gov/35807892/.
https://pubmed.ncbi.nlm.nih.gov/32640566/. https://pubmed.ncbi.nlm.nih.gov/31272234/.
1046. Articles:
https://www.ncbi.nlm.nih.gov/pmc/articles/PMC10459106/#:~:text=Agin%20et%20al.,pediatric%
20study%20group%20%5B40%5D. https://www.ncbi.nlm.nih.gov/pmc/articles/PMC6308038/.
https://bmcgastroenterol.biomedcentral.com/articles/10.1186/s12876-016-0543-z.
https://journals.lww.com/ajg/fulltext/2016/10001/a_neglected_field_of_peptic_ulcer_disease_thera
py_.1136.aspx.
1047. Articles: https://pubmed.ncbi.nlm.nih.gov/3028346/.
https://pubmed.ncbi.nlm.nih.gov/23093388/. https://pubmed.ncbi.nlm.nih.gov/29431349/.
1048. Articles: https://pubmed.ncbi.nlm.nih.gov/34717822/.
https://pubmed.ncbi.nlm.nih.gov/37380191/. https://pubmed.ncbi.nlm.nih.gov/38048800/.
https://pubmed.ncbi.nlm.nih.gov/30977444/.
1049. Related articles: https://pubmed.ncbi.nlm.nih.gov/4348890/.

1050. Articles:
https://www.proquest.com/openview/44c3ce1fb901382e8ee779da0a5d96da/1?pq-origsite=gscholar&cbl=4991861.
https://jarem.org/articles/the-effects-of-vitamin-d-in-patients-with-subacromial-impingement-syndrome/doi/jarem.2019.2126.
1051. Articles: https://pubmed.ncbi.nlm.nih.gov/15727633/.
https://curology.com/blog/fact-vs-fiction-vitamin-d-and-acne/.
1052. Articles: https://pubmed.ncbi.nlm.nih.gov/12710640/.
https://pubmed.ncbi.nlm.nih.gov/23600989/. https://pubmed.ncbi.nlm.nih.gov/6966389/.
https://pubmed.ncbi.nlm.nih.gov/25019937/. https://pubmed.ncbi.nlm.nih.gov/10434505/.
https://pubmed.ncbi.nlm.nih.gov/10459231/.
1053. Articles:
https://www.css.ch/en/private-customers/my-health/health-glossary/conditions/complex-regional-pain-syndrome-crps.html.
https://www.reumatologiaclinica.org/en-complex-regional-pain-syndrome-type-articulo-resumen-S2173574317300199.
1054. Tragically, there can be little doubt that many people who commit, or attempt to commit, suicide are simply deficient in vitamin D. L.S. Articles: https://pubmed.ncbi.nlm.nih.gov/32388454/.
https://pubmed.ncbi.nlm.nih.gov/37049606/. https://pubmed.ncbi.nlm.nih.gov/37881417/.
https://pubmed.ncbi.nlm.nih.gov/26681234/.
https://journals.plos.org/plosone/article?id=10.1371/journal.pone.0279166.
https://www.webmd.com/vitamins-and-supplements/what-to-know-about-vitamin-d-and-mental-health.
1055. Bowles, p. 62. Articles: https://pubmed.ncbi.nlm.nih.gov/28615360/.
https://pubmed.ncbi.nlm.nih.gov/28941472/.
1056. Article: https://pubmed.ncbi.nlm.nih.gov/29393614/.
1057. Articles: https://www.ncbi.nlm.nih.gov/pmc/articles/PMC8318784/.
https://www.healthline.com/nutrition/vitamin-d-coronavirus.
1058. Articles: https://pubmed.ncbi.nlm.nih.gov/29669433/.
https://pubmed.ncbi.nlm.nih.gov/33738914/.
1059. Articles: https://pubmed.ncbi.nlm.nih.gov/15400837/.
https://pubmed.ncbi.nlm.nih.gov/26575832/. https://pubmed.ncbi.nlm.nih.gov/23227442/.
1060. Articles: https://www.exercise.com/learn/can-low-vitamin-d-cause-swollen-lymph-nodes/.
https://www.ncbi.nlm.nih.gov/pmc/articles/PMC5031886/.
1061. Article: https://pubmed.ncbi.nlm.nih.gov/46514/.
1062. Articles: https://pubmed.ncbi.nlm.nih.gov/32518053/.
https://pubmed.ncbi.nlm.nih.gov/27294593/. https://pubmed.ncbi.nlm.nih.gov/34830503/.
1063. Article: https://pubmed.ncbi.nlm.nih.gov/11952079/. Related article:
https://pubmed.ncbi.nlm.nih.gov/30567100/.
1064. Articles: https://www.ncbi.nlm.nih.gov/pmc/articles/PMC4922356/.
https://www.tandfonline.com/doi/full/10.1080/16089677.2023.2178155.
https://pubmed.ncbi.nlm.nih.gov/34522473/. https://pubmed.ncbi.nlm.nih.gov/22218780/.
https://pubmed.ncbi.nlm.nih.gov/36188735/.
1065. Articles: https://pubmed.ncbi.nlm.nih.gov/37123896/.
https://pubmed.ncbi.nlm.nih.gov/33301353/. https://pubmed.ncbi.nlm.nih.gov/31877381/.
https://pubmed.ncbi.nlm.nih.gov/27611796/.
1066. Vitamin D deficiency has been linked to autoimmune-inflammatory diseases like lupus. Because lupus patients must avoid exposure to the sun, adequate vitamin D from other sources is imperative for good health. Weiss, p. 221. See also Dowd and Stafford, pp. 157-159. Articles:
https://pubmed.ncbi.nlm.nih.gov/35648165/. https://pubmed.ncbi.nlm.nih.gov/37189455/.
https://pubmed.ncbi.nlm.nih.gov/29108830/.
1067. Articles: https://pubmed.ncbi.nlm.nih.gov/36813139/.
https://pubmed.ncbi.nlm.nih.gov/32563782/. https://pubmed.ncbi.nlm.nih.gov/36235561/.
1068. Articles: https://pubmed.ncbi.nlm.nih.gov/26808323/.
https://pubmed.ncbi.nlm.nih.gov/28531358/. https://pubmed.ncbi.nlm.nih.gov/29393614/.
https://pubmed.ncbi.nlm.nih.gov/37510843/.
1069. Articles: https://pubmed.ncbi.nlm.nih.gov/26661754/.
https://pubmed.ncbi.nlm.nih.gov/30481900/. https://pubmed.ncbi.nlm.nih.gov/38598024/.
https://pubmed.ncbi.nlm.nih.gov/34692838/.

1070. Articles: https://pubmed.ncbi.nlm.nih.gov/23482610/.
https://pubmed.ncbi.nlm.nih.gov/24036395/.

1071. Articles: https://www.mdpi.com/2072-6643/12/4/984.
https://pubmed.ncbi.nlm.nih.gov/32252288/.

1072. Vitamin D has been found to strengthen resistance to tuberculosis. *Food and Nutrition*, p. 30.
Articles: https://pubmed.ncbi.nlm.nih.gov/32706534/.
https://pubmed.ncbi.nlm.nih.gov/35352542/. https://pubmed.ncbi.nlm.nih.gov/35409219/.
https://pubmed.ncbi.nlm.nih.gov/19386033/. https://pubmed.ncbi.nlm.nih.gov/26058744/.

1073. Related articles: https://pubmed.ncbi.nlm.nih.gov/35682491/.
https://pubmed.ncbi.nlm.nih.gov/32384728/.

1074. Related articles: https://pubmed.ncbi.nlm.nih.gov/37732453/.
https://pubmed.ncbi.nlm.nih.gov/32771307/.

1075. Articles: https://pubmed.ncbi.nlm.nih.gov/32084549/.
https://pubmed.ncbi.nlm.nih.gov/32438644/.

1076. Articles: https://pubmed.ncbi.nlm.nih.gov/30344276/.
https://pubmed.ncbi.nlm.nih.gov/37273020/. https://pubmed.ncbi.nlm.nih.gov/37966493/.

1077. Articles: https://www.ncbi.nlm.nih.gov/pmc/articles/PMC7285165/.
https://www.smilesbyshields.com/vitamin-d-deficiency-and-dental-health/.

1078. Articles: https://pubmed.ncbi.nlm.nih.gov/36082312/.
https://pubmed.ncbi.nlm.nih.gov/29332745/.

1079. Article: https://pubmed.ncbi.nlm.nih.gov/35852202/.

1080. Articles: https://pubmed.ncbi.nlm.nih.gov/34067977/.
https://pubmed.ncbi.nlm.nih.gov/37242266/. https://pubmed.ncbi.nlm.nih.gov/28030821/.
https://pubmed.ncbi.nlm.nih.gov/29765521/. https://pubmed.ncbi.nlm.nih.gov/24419359/.

1081. Articles: https://pubmed.ncbi.nlm.nih.gov/32341213/.
https://www.frontiersin.org/journals/endocrinology/articles/10.3389/fendo.2022.960222/full.
https://www.ncbi.nlm.nih.gov/pmc/articles/PMC10518189/.
https://sciencenews.dk/en/vitamin-d-increases-testosterone-production.

1082. Articles: https://pubmed.ncbi.nlm.nih.gov/37354510/.
https://pubmed.ncbi.nlm.nih.gov/36381723/. https://pubmed.ncbi.nlm.nih.gov/29075541/.

1083. Articles: https://pubmed.ncbi.nlm.nih.gov/33423084/.
https://pubmed.ncbi.nlm.nih.gov/24106607/. https://pubmed.ncbi.nlm.nih.gov/36763189/.
https://pubmed.ncbi.nlm.nih.gov/38132240/.

1084. Articles: https://pubmed.ncbi.nlm.nih.gov/31203812/.
https://pubmed.ncbi.nlm.nih.gov/37145323/. https://pubmed.ncbi.nlm.nih.gov/32287103/.
https://pubmed.ncbi.nlm.nih.gov/23556539/. https://pubmed.ncbi.nlm.nih.gov/27312171/.

1085. Articles: https://pubmed.ncbi.nlm.nih.gov/23256106/.
https://pubmed.ncbi.nlm.nih.gov/33100166/. https://pubmed.ncbi.nlm.nih.gov/38590944/.
https://pubmed.ncbi.nlm.nih.gov/26934010/. https://pubmed.ncbi.nlm.nih.gov/38144238/.

1086. Articles: https://pubmed.ncbi.nlm.nih.gov/33719687/.
https://pubmed.ncbi.nlm.nih.gov/36876384/.

1087. Articles: https://pubmed.ncbi.nlm.nih.gov/26860322/.
https://pubmed.ncbi.nlm.nih.gov/38375518/. https://pubmed.ncbi.nlm.nih.gov/38373939/.

1088. Articles: https://pubmed.ncbi.nlm.nih.gov/36362448/.
https://pubmed.ncbi.nlm.nih.gov/28895880/. https://pubmed.ncbi.nlm.nih.gov/30086436/.

1089. Articles: https://pubmed.ncbi.nlm.nih.gov/33679732/.
https://pubmed.ncbi.nlm.nih.gov/28895880/. https://pubmed.ncbi.nlm.nih.gov/36835005/.

1090. Related articles: https://pubmed.ncbi.nlm.nih.gov/22961293/.
https://pubmed.ncbi.nlm.nih.gov/26620753/. https://pubmed.ncbi.nlm.nih.gov/38450273/.
https://pubmed.ncbi.nlm.nih.gov/30033803/. https://pubmed.ncbi.nlm.nih.gov/33266477/.

1091. Article: https://pubmed.ncbi.nlm.nih.gov/29314669/.

1092. Related article: https://www.ncbi.nlm.nih.gov/pmc/articles/PMC9220304/.

1093. Articles: https://pubmed.ncbi.nlm.nih.gov/33476988/.
https://www.ijord.com/index.php/ijord/article/view/1103.
https://www.producer.com/livestock/vitamins-solve-ringworm-problem/#:~:text=Healthy%20skin
%20is%20a%20great,which%20helps%20kill%20this%20organism. Related:
https://www.healthline.com/health/fungal-infection/which-vitamin-deficiency-causes-fungal-infection.

1094. Articles: https://www.ijord.com/index.php/ijord/article/view/1103.

1095. Article: https://www.ncbi.nlm.nih.gov/pmc/articles/PMC7733373/.

1096. Article:
https://omegaquant.com/can-low-vitamin-d-cause-neuropathy/#:~:text=BLOG%3A%20How%20to
%20Choose%20the,the%20hands%20and%2For%20feet.

1097. Articles: https://pubmed.ncbi.nlm.nih.gov/36980345/.
https://pubmed.ncbi.nlm.nih.gov/37636653/. https://pubmed.ncbi.nlm.nih.gov/34407088/.
https://pubmed.ncbi.nlm.nih.gov/38545900/. https://pubmed.ncbi.nlm.nih.gov/31356390/.

1098. Bowles, p. 55. Article: https://pubmed.ncbi.nlm.nih.gov/34188748/.

1099. Articles: https://pubmed.ncbi.nlm.nih.gov/36974865/.
https://pubmed.ncbi.nlm.nih.gov/35886596/. https://pubmed.ncbi.nlm.nih.gov/37198277/.
https://pubmed.ncbi.nlm.nih.gov/32689892/.

1100. Articles:
https://www.smilesbyshields.com/vitamin-d-deficiency-and-dental-health/#:~:text=Lack%20of%20vi
tamin%20D%20can,who%20received%20vitamin%20D%20supplements.
https://bmcoralhealth.biomedcentral.com/articles/10.1186/s12903-023-03422-z.
https://pubmed.ncbi.nlm.nih.gov/32438644/.

1101. Article:
https://www.periodonticsnaples.com/3-vitamin-deficiencies-that-affect-tooth-and-gum-health.
https://www.everlywell.com/blog/vitamin-d/can-low-vitamin-d-affect-your-teeth/.

1102. Article: https://www.health.com/mind-body/vitamin-d-health-risks.

1103. Articles: https://pubmed.ncbi.nlm.nih.gov/37569267/.
https://pubmed.ncbi.nlm.nih.gov/37325365/. https://pubmed.ncbi.nlm.nih.gov/35685731/.
https://pubmed.ncbi.nlm.nih.gov/38385037/. https://pubmed.ncbi.nlm.nih.gov/38396228/.
https://pubmed.ncbi.nlm.nih.gov/29132463/.
https://www.ncbi.nlm.nih.gov/pmc/articles/PMC10267821/#:~:text=Pooled%20prevalence%20of
%20vitD%20deficiency,%2C%20I2%20%3D%2097%25. Related article:
https://www.ncbi.nlm.nih.gov/pmc/articles/PMC6716592/.

1104. Related articles:
https://www.healio.com/news/endocrinology/20190226/ht-does-not-alter-vitamin-d-levels-in-transg
ender-adults#:~:text=At%20baseline%2C%2041%25%20of%20transgender,were%20considered%20v
itamin%20D%20deficient. https://academic.oup.com/jcem/article/104/7/2728/5342944.
https://pubmed.ncbi.nlm.nih.gov/31573999/. https://pubmed.ncbi.nlm.nih.gov/34497118/.
https://pubmed.ncbi.nlm.nih.gov/37450195/. https://pubmed.ncbi.nlm.nih.gov/14515001/.
https://pubmed.ncbi.nlm.nih.gov/38343146/. https://pubmed.ncbi.nlm.nih.gov/25377496/.
https://link.springer.com/article/10.1007/s40618-023-02156-7.
https://pubmed.ncbi.nlm.nih.gov/34497118/.

1105. Related articles:
https://www.healio.com/news/endocrinology/20190226/ht-does-not-alter-vitamin-d-levels-in-transg
ender-adults#:~:text=At%20baseline%2C%2041%25%20of%20transgender,were%20considered%20v
itamin%20D%20deficient. https://academic.oup.com/jcem/article/104/7/2728/5342944.
https://pubmed.ncbi.nlm.nih.gov/31573999/. https://pubmed.ncbi.nlm.nih.gov/34497118/.
https://pubmed.ncbi.nlm.nih.gov/37450195/. https://pubmed.ncbi.nlm.nih.gov/14515001/.
https://pubmed.ncbi.nlm.nih.gov/38343146/. https://pubmed.ncbi.nlm.nih.gov/25377496/.
https://link.springer.com/article/10.1007/s40618-023-02156-7.
https://pubmed.ncbi.nlm.nih.gov/34497118/.

1106. Related articles: https://pubmed.ncbi.nlm.nih.gov/22961293/.
https://pubmed.ncbi.nlm.nih.gov/26620753/. https://pubmed.ncbi.nlm.nih.gov/38450273/.
https://pubmed.ncbi.nlm.nih.gov/30033803/. https://pubmed.ncbi.nlm.nih.gov/33266477/.

1107. Articles:
https://www.neurology.org/doi/10.1212/NXI.0000000000000004#:~:text=Kimbrough%20et%20a
l.%2C%20along%20with,was%20also%20abnormal%20or%20not.
https://jamanetwork.com/journals/jamaneurology/fullarticle/1108016.
https://pubmed.ncbi.nlm.nih.gov/22083799/.
https://www.nutraingredients-usa.com/Article/2011/11/15/Low-vitamin-D-Levels-linked-to-spinal-c
ord-inflammatory-disease.
https://wearesrna.org/resources/association-between-low-vitamin-d-levels-and-recurrent-inflammator
y-spinal-cord-disease/.

1108. Articles: https://pubmed.ncbi.nlm.nih.gov/36820164/.
https://pubmed.ncbi.nlm.nih.gov/35741675/. https://pubmed.ncbi.nlm.nih.gov/32908795/.
https://pubmed.ncbi.nlm.nih.gov/33983694/.

1109. Articles:
https://www.researchgate.net/publication/339913302_Paediatric_gastric_trichobezoar_the_Rapunzel
_syndrome_A_report_of_two_cases.
https://www.anncaserep.com/open-access/association-of-pediatric-rapunzel-syndrome-with-proteinlos
ing-enteropathybr-nbsp-6030.pdf.
https://www.degruyter.com/document/doi/10.1515/med-2020-0243/html?lang=en.
https://www.emjreviews.com/dermatology/article/trichotillomania-with-giant-gastric-trichobezoar-in
-a-female-child-a-case-report/.

1110. Related articles: https://pubmed.ncbi.nlm.nih.gov/38346419/.
https://pubmed.ncbi.nlm.nih.gov/27521899/. https://pubmed.ncbi.nlm.nih.gov/28571565/.

1111. Article: https://pubmed.ncbi.nlm.nih.gov/28426188/.

1112. Articles: https://pubmed.ncbi.nlm.nih.gov/34553483/.
https://pubmed.ncbi.nlm.nih.gov/31942278/. https://pubmed.ncbi.nlm.nih.gov/30649027/.

1113. Articles: https://pubmed.ncbi.nlm.nih.gov/30334198/.
https://pubmed.ncbi.nlm.nih.gov/32246668/.

1114. Possible related articles: https://pubmed.ncbi.nlm.nih.gov/36381723/.
https://pubmed.ncbi.nlm.nih.gov/22251708/. https://pubmed.ncbi.nlm.nih.gov/29982185/.

1115. Vitamin D has been found to strengthen resistance to tuberculosis. *Food and Nutrition*, p. 30.
Articles: https://pubmed.ncbi.nlm.nih.gov/32706534/.
https://pubmed.ncbi.nlm.nih.gov/35352542/. https://pubmed.ncbi.nlm.nih.gov/35409219/.
https://pubmed.ncbi.nlm.nih.gov/19386033/. https://pubmed.ncbi.nlm.nih.gov/26058744/.

1116. Articles: https://pubmed.ncbi.nlm.nih.gov/38846332/.
https://pubmed.ncbi.nlm.nih.gov/9192275/. https://pubmed.ncbi.nlm.nih.gov/31338111/.
https://pubmed.ncbi.nlm.nih.gov/6603629/. https://pubmed.ncbi.nlm.nih.gov/36331254/.

1117. Articles: https://pubmed.ncbi.nlm.nih.gov/36511653/.
https://pubmed.ncbi.nlm.nih.gov/30775554/. https://pubmed.ncbi.nlm.nih.gov/32504138/.
https://pubmed.ncbi.nlm.nih.gov/29021995/. https://pubmed.ncbi.nlm.nih.gov/28703220/.

1118. Related articles: https://www.dshs.texas.gov/citrullinemia.
https://pubmed.ncbi.nlm.nih.gov/3067584/.

1119. Articles: https://pubmed.ncbi.nlm.nih.gov/38004239/.
https://pubmed.ncbi.nlm.nih.gov/33396382/. https://pubmed.ncbi.nlm.nih.gov/30384373/.
https://pubmed.ncbi.nlm.nih.gov/34075433/.

1120. Article:
https://www.frontiersin.org/journals/nutrition/articles/10.3389/fnut.2023.1132191/full.

1121. Related articles: https://www.btf-thyroid.org/vitamin-d-and-thyroid-disease.
https://www.ncbi.nlm.nih.gov/pmc/articles/PMC3921055/.
https://www.ncbi.nlm.nih.gov/pmc/articles/PMC9964959/.
https://thyroiduk.org/if-you-are-hypothyroid/the-importance-of-vitamins-and-minerals-hypo/vitamin-
d/. https://pubmed.ncbi.nlm.nih.gov/28315909/. https://pubmed.ncbi.nlm.nih.gov/34064075/.
https://pubmed.ncbi.nlm.nih.gov/35440339/.

1122. Articles: https://pubmed.ncbi.nlm.nih.gov/20386089/.
https://pubmed.ncbi.nlm.nih.gov/26096436/.
https://academic.oup.com/nutritionreviews/article-abstract/82/2/166/7169182.
https://www.ncbi.nlm.nih.gov/pmc/articles/PMC8932030/.

1123. Articles: https://pubmed.ncbi.nlm.nih.gov/37321901/.
https://pubmed.ncbi.nlm.nih.gov/36370297/. https://pubmed.ncbi.nlm.nih.gov/34080787/.
https://pubmed.ncbi.nlm.nih.gov/29602840/. https://pubmed.ncbi.nlm.nih.gov/30972950/.
https://pubmed.ncbi.nlm.nih.gov/25359617/.

1124. Articles: https://pubmed.ncbi.nlm.nih.gov/34491371/.
https://pubmed.ncbi.nlm.nih.gov/32387293/. https://pubmed.ncbi.nlm.nih.gov/32479701/.
https://pubmed.ncbi.nlm.nih.gov/32001360/.

1125. Articles: https://pubmed.ncbi.nlm.nih.gov/28749951/.
https://pubmed.ncbi.nlm.nih.gov/30814089/.

1126. Articles: https://academic.oup.com/nutritionreviews/article-abstract/82/2/166/7169182.
https://ufhealth.org/conditions-and-treatments/hypervitaminosis-d.
https://austinurologyinstitute.com/blog/vitamin-d-and-bladder-urinary-tract-health/.

1127. Articles: https://pubmed.ncbi.nlm.nih.gov/32032687/.
https://pubmed.ncbi.nlm.nih.gov/30136085/. https://pubmed.ncbi.nlm.nih.gov/29562593/.
https://pubmed.ncbi.nlm.nih.gov/34959915/.

1128. Articles: https://pubmed.ncbi.nlm.nih.gov/29064205/.
https://pubmed.ncbi.nlm.nih.gov/22171613/. https://pubmed.ncbi.nlm.nih.gov/25155458/.
1129. Articles: https://pubmed.ncbi.nlm.nih.gov/33504114/.
https://pubmed.ncbi.nlm.nih.gov/30011902/. https://pubmed.ncbi.nlm.nih.gov/33670322/.
1130. Articles: https://pubmed.ncbi.nlm.nih.gov/36150919/.
https://pubmed.ncbi.nlm.nih.gov/23824422/. https://pubmed.ncbi.nlm.nih.gov/30172168/.
1131. Articles:
https://www.ncbi.nlm.nih.gov/pmc/articles/PMC5713297/#:~:text=Both%20vitamin%20D%20an
d%20its,ovarian%2C%20cervical%20and%20vulvar%20cancer.
https://pubmed.ncbi.nlm.nih.gov/29113037/. https://pubmed.ncbi.nlm.nih.gov/24605180/.
1132. Articles: https://pubmed.ncbi.nlm.nih.gov/29897832/.
https://pubmed.ncbi.nlm.nih.gov/17368903/.
1133. Articles:
https://www.frontiersin.org/journals/nutrition/articles/10.3389/fnut.2022.1016592/full.
https://www.ncbi.nlm.nih.gov/pmc/articles/PMC4525405/.
https://cdn.mdedge.com/files/s3fs-public/Document/September-2017/086010039.pdf.
1134. Articles: https://www.ncbi.nlm.nih.gov/pmc/articles/PMC4525405/.
https://bmcinfectdis.biomedcentral.com/articles/10.1186/s12879-023-08120-3.
1135. Articles: https://www.healthylife.com.au/learn/chicken-pox.
https://pubmed.ncbi.nlm.nih.gov/25487609/. https://pubmed.ncbi.nlm.nih.gov/38423817/.
https://www.ukbiobank.ac.uk/enable-your-research/approved-research/association-between-serum-vi
tamin-d-deficiency-and-the-risk-of-herpes-zoster-a-longitudinal-uk-biobank-study.
1136. Articles: https://pubmed.ncbi.nlm.nih.gov/13891349/.
https://www.theprivateclinic.co.uk/blog/are-varicose-veins-caused-by-a-vitamin-deficiency/#:~:text
=Vitamin%20D%20and%20Varicose%20Veins&text=Vitamin%20D%20also%20works%20to,issues%2
0such%20as%20varicose%20veins.
https://www.veinvascular.com/vein/these-vitamins-can-prevent-varicose-vein-surgery/.
1137. Articles: https://pubmed.ncbi.nlm.nih.gov/17218831/.
https://pubmed.ncbi.nlm.nih.gov/20795937/.
1138. Articles: https://pubmed.ncbi.nlm.nih.gov/36874269/.
https://pubmed.ncbi.nlm.nih.gov/35277211/. https://pubmed.ncbi.nlm.nih.gov/33454206/.
https://pubmed.ncbi.nlm.nih.gov/33340057/.
1139. Articles:
https://www.nutri-facts.org/en_US/news/articles/an-insufficient-vitamin-d-supply-may-be-related-to
-vein-thrombos.html. https://www.ncbi.nlm.nih.gov/pmc/articles/PMC4069050/.
https://us.supersmart.com/en/blog/cardiovascular/phlebitis-what-to-eat-what-not-to-eat-s626.
1140. Articles: https://pubmed.ncbi.nlm.nih.gov/22481708/.
https://pubmed.ncbi.nlm.nih.gov/31903952/. https://pubmed.ncbi.nlm.nih.gov/32319144/.
1141. Articles: https://pubmed.ncbi.nlm.nih.gov/33307795/.
https://pubmed.ncbi.nlm.nih.gov/27786545/. https://pubmed.ncbi.nlm.nih.gov/27775457/.
https://pubmed.ncbi.nlm.nih.gov/38770629/.
1142. Articles: https://pubmed.ncbi.nlm.nih.gov/32759193/.
https://pubmed.ncbi.nlm.nih.gov/38474817/. https://pubmed.ncbi.nlm.nih.gov/32767116/.
1143. Articles: https://pubmed.ncbi.nlm.nih.gov/38529069/.
https://pubmed.ncbi.nlm.nih.gov/12455400/. https://pubmed.ncbi.nlm.nih.gov/8148393/.
https://pubmed.ncbi.nlm.nih.gov/34137176/.
1144. Article: https://www.ncbi.nlm.nih.gov/pmc/articles/PMC4511535/.
1145. Articles: https://pubmed.ncbi.nlm.nih.gov/34322844/.
https://pubmed.ncbi.nlm.nih.gov/32679784/. https://pubmed.ncbi.nlm.nih.gov/37686873/.
https://pubmed.ncbi.nlm.nih.gov/38777416/. https://pubmed.ncbi.nlm.nih.gov/32967126/.
1146. Articles: https://pubmed.ncbi.nlm.nih.gov/32679784/.
https://pubmed.ncbi.nlm.nih.gov/35507293/. https://pubmed.ncbi.nlm.nih.gov/26035247/.
1147. Articles:
https://versanthealth.com/blog/how-can-vitamin-d-deficiency-negatively-impact-eye-health/#:~:text
=Vitamin%20D%20is%20also%20critical,on%20eyesight%20in%20many%20ways.
https://www.healthline.com/health/eye-health/macular-degeneration-vitamin-d.
https://doctorsclinichouston.com/general-health/vitamin-d3-and-eye-health/.
https://www.aao.org/eyenet/article/vitamin-d-and-ocular-diseases.

1148. Articles: https://pubmed.ncbi.nlm.nih.gov/28994020/.
https://pubmed.ncbi.nlm.nih.gov/36558443/. https://pubmed.ncbi.nlm.nih.gov/35871394/.
https://pubmed.ncbi.nlm.nih.gov/36254395/.
1149. Articles: https://www.medscape.com/viewarticle/755046?form=fpf.
https://pubmed.ncbi.nlm.nih.gov/37661522/. https://pubmed.ncbi.nlm.nih.gov/28772303/.
https://www.ncbi.nlm.nih.gov/pmc/articles/PMC7774915/.
1150. Articles: https://pubmed.ncbi.nlm.nih.gov/30813930/.
https://pubmed.ncbi.nlm.nih.gov/27599751/. https://pubmed.ncbi.nlm.nih.gov/15658149/.
1151. Articles: https://pubmed.ncbi.nlm.nih.gov/28029003/.
https://pubmed.ncbi.nlm.nih.gov/35416396/. https://pubmed.ncbi.nlm.nih.gov/30519274/.
https://pubmed.ncbi.nlm.nih.gov/35420222/. https://pubmed.ncbi.nlm.nih.gov/35646274/.
1152. Articles:
https://www.ncbi.nlm.nih.gov/pmc/articles/PMC5713297/#:~:text=Both%20vitamin%20D%20an
d%20its,ovarian%2C%20cervical%20and%20vulvar%20cancer.
https://pubmed.ncbi.nlm.nih.gov/29113037/. https://pubmed.ncbi.nlm.nih.gov/24605180/.
1153. Articles: https://www.medicinenet.com/what_causes_delay_in_walking_in_babies/article.htm.
https://www.lebonheur.org/blogs/practical-parenting/vitamin-d-supplement-recommended-for-all-inf
ants#:~:text=While%20early%20vitamin%20D%20deficiency,spot%20on%20an%20infant's%20head.
https://www.ncbi.nlm.nih.gov/pmc/articles/PMC6586450/.
https://www.healthline.com/nutrition/vitamin-d-deficiency-in-kids-and-teens.
1154. Articles: https://pubmed.ncbi.nlm.nih.gov/33860625/.
https://pubmed.ncbi.nlm.nih.gov/26294740/. https://pubmed.ncbi.nlm.nih.gov/32118375/.
https://pubmed.ncbi.nlm.nih.gov/31925891/.
1155. Articles: https://pubmed.ncbi.nlm.nih.gov/15182797/.
https://www.careatc.com/improving-health/the-link-between-shoulder-pain-and-vitamin-d-deficiency.
https://pubmed.ncbi.nlm.nih.gov/30321335/. https://pubmed.ncbi.nlm.nih.gov/6387576/.
https://pubmed.ncbi.nlm.nih.gov/33390486/. https://pubmed.ncbi.nlm.nih.gov/7014108/.
https://annalsmedres.org/index.php/aomr/article/view/448.
https://www.tampabay.com/news/health/Mayo-Clinic-Q-A-treating-frozen-shoulder-calcium-supple
ments-versus-exercise_165896098/.
https://www.businessinsider.com/guides/health/treatments/frozen-shoulder.
1156. Article:
https://www.webmd.com/vitamins-and-supplements/what-to-know-about-vitamin-d-and-mental-healt
h.
1157. Article:
https://www.webmd.com/vitamins-and-supplements/what-to-know-about-vitamin-d-and-mental-healt
h.
1158. Article:
https://www.semanticscholar.org/paper/A-case-of-weill-marchesani-syndrome-with-a-novel-d-Y%C4
%B1ld%C4%B1r%C4%B1m/6ccbb9e51169891f780a909d26c71d41052f08ab.
1159. Article: https://pubmed.ncbi.nlm.nih.gov/11952079/.
1160. Articles:
https://www.mayoclinic.org/diseases-conditions/whipples-disease/diagnosis-treatment/drc-20378950
. https://www.ncbi.nlm.nih.gov/pmc/articles/PMC3703430/.
https://www.healthline.com/health/whipples-disease.
https://www.sciencedirect.com/science/article/pii/S120197122100271X.
1161. Article:
https://www.asarchcenter.com/blog/which-vitamin-deficiency-causes-white-spots-on-skin/. Related
article:
https://mydiagnostics.in/blogs/nutritional/heres-how-to-identify-vitamin-deficiency-small-white-spots-
on-skin.
1162. Articles:
https://www.ncbi.nlm.nih.gov/pmc/articles/PMC4760950/#:~:text=Vitamin%20D3%20(VD3,pert
ussis%20infection. https://journals.plos.org/plosone/article?id=10.1371/journal.pone.0149576.
1163. Article: https://pubmed.ncbi.nlm.nih.gov/35617449/.
1164. Article: https://pubmed.ncbi.nlm.nih.gov/20301427/.
1165. Articles: https://pubmed.ncbi.nlm.nih.gov/24572979/.
https://pubmed.ncbi.nlm.nih.gov/33856702/.
1166. Articles: https://pubmed.ncbi.nlm.nih.gov/11373341/.
https://pubmed.ncbi.nlm.nih.gov/11050081/.

1167. Related articles: https://pubmed.ncbi.nlm.nih.gov/37415038/. https://pubmed.ncbi.nlm.nih.gov/32228506/.

1168. Caution: Vitamin D production in the skin can drop severely during the cold months. Steps should be taken to counteract this problem. *Bottom Line's 2021 Health Breakthroughs*, p. 304.

1169. Article: https://www.webmd.com/vitamins-and-supplements/what-to-know-about-vitamin-d-and-mental-health.

1170. Articles: https://www.ncbi.nlm.nih.gov/pmc/articles/PMC9220304/. https://link.springer.com/referenceworkentry/10.1007/978-1-60761-219-3_97. https://onlinelibrary.wiley.com/doi/10.1002/clc.22329.

1171. Related article: https://pubmed.ncbi.nlm.nih.gov/36133901/.

1172. Article: https://www.ncbi.nlm.nih.gov/pmc/articles/PMC4511535/.

1173. Articles: https://pubmed.ncbi.nlm.nih.gov/32654618/. https://www.woundsource.com/blog/there-association-between-vitamin-d-and-wound-healing. https://www.healthline.com/nutrition/vitamin-d-deficiency-symptoms#:~:text=Symptoms%20of%20vitamin%20D%20deficiency%20may%20include%20fatigue%2C%20frequent%20illness,dietary%20changes%20or%20taking%20supplements. https://whitneyrehab.com/why-you-need-to-avoid-low-vitamin-d-levels/.

1174. Articles: https://pubmed.ncbi.nlm.nih.gov/20301621/. https://pubmed.ncbi.nlm.nih.gov/26643206/. https://pubmed.ncbi.nlm.nih.gov/3794931/. https://pubmed.ncbi.nlm.nih.gov/16121806/.

1175. Articles: https://pubmed.ncbi.nlm.nih.gov/37150017/. https://pubmed.ncbi.nlm.nih.gov/37847693/. https://www.sciencedirect.com/science/article/abs/pii/S1567576923005532.

1176. Article: https://pubmed.ncbi.nlm.nih.gov/

1177. See Webpage: https://www.cdc.gov/obesity/basics/consequences.html.

1178. See Webpage: https://www.cdc.gov/tobacco/about/index.html.

1179. See Webpage: https://www.cdc.gov/alcohol/about-alcohol-use/index.html.

1180. See Webpage: https://www.cdc.gov/nutrition/data-statistics/sugar-sweetened-beverages-intake.html#:~:text=Frequently%20drinking%20sugar%2Dsweetened%20beverages,gout%2C%0a%20type%20of%20arthritis.

1181. See Webpage: https://www.ncbi.nlm.nih.gov/pmc/articles/PMC1804190/.

1182. See articles: https://www.ncbi.nlm.nih.gov/pmc/articles/PMC8932957/. https://www.ncbi.nlm.nih.gov/pmc/articles/PMC9571750/. https://pubmed.ncbi.nlm.nih.gov/29699509/. https://pubmed.ncbi.nlm.nih.gov/33826120/. https://pubmed.ncbi.nlm.nih.gov/36257717/. https://pubmed.ncbi.nlm.nih.gov/36771239/.

1183. See articles: https://sallyknorton.com/oxalate-science/. https://www.webmd.com/diet/foods-high-in-oxalates. https://pubmed.ncbi.nlm.nih.gov/24393738/.

1184. See articles: https://gundryhealth.com/health-dangers-of-lectins/. https://www.healthline.com/nutrition/foods-high-in-lectins#TOC_TITLE_HDR_7. https://www.webmd.com/diet/foods-high-in-lectins.

1185. See articles: https://www.webmd.com/diet/what-to-know-about-nightshade-vegetables. https://www.arthritis.org/health-wellness/healthy-living/nutrition/anti-inflammatory/how-nightshades-affect-arthritis. https://www.healthline.com/health/most-nutritious-nightshade-plants.

1186. See e.g., video: "The Longevity and Brain Benefits of Vigorous Exercise," by Dr. Rhonda Patrick. YouTube channel: FoundMyFitness.

1187. For more on this topic see my books *Jesus and the Law of Attraction* and *The Bible and the Law of Attraction*.

1188. See video: "The Unique Benefits of Using Vitamin D and K2 Combined." YouTube channel: Dr. Eric Berg DC. Note: Always consult and work with a licensed physician when taking vitamin and mineral supplements. L.S.

1189. Video: "#1 Vitamin D Danger You Absolutely Must Know!" YouTube channel: Dr. Sten Ekberg.

1190. See https://www.govinfo.gov/content/pkg/GPO-CRECB-1973-pt1/pdf/GPO-CRECB-1973-pt1-1-2.pdf, p. 53.

1191. Rep. Hosmer's commonsense bill "would prohibit the Food and Drug Administration from limiting dosage or ordering warning labels on any 'food supplement' that is not 'intrinsically dangerous to health.'" Congressional Hearing, p. 688.

1192. Congressional Hearing, pp. 603-605.
1193. Congressional Hearing, pp. 756-757.
1194. Congressional Hearing, pp. 772-773.
1195. Congressional Hearing, pp. 793-794.
1196. Congressional Hearing, pp. 794-796.
1197. Congressional Hearing, pp. 797-798.

BIBLIOGRAPHY

And Suggested Reading

Acton, Q. Ashton (ed.). *Advances in Vitamin D Deficiency Research and Treatment.* Atlanta, GA: Scholarly Editions, 2012.

Altshul, Sara, and Pamela Hops. *Kitchen Cabinet Cures: 1,001 Homemade Remedies for Your Health.* Pleasantville, NY: Reader's Digest, 2010.

Attkisson, Sharyl. *Follow the Science: How Big Pharma Misleads, Obscures, and Prevails.* New York: Harper, 2024.

Bottom Line's 2021 Health Breakthroughs. Stamford, CT: Bottom Line Inc., 2020.

Bowles, Jeff T. *The Miraculous Results of Extremely High Doses of the Sunshine Hormone Vitamin D3.* Troutdale, OR: Jeff T. Bowles Publishing, no date.

Brown, Susan E. *Better Bones, Better Body : Beyond Estrogen and Calcium.* New York: McGraw Hill, 2000.

Busch, Felicia. *Smart Nutrition: The Essential Vitamin, Mineral and Supplement Reference Guide.* Minnetonka, MN: National Health and Wellness Club, 2004.

Cannell, John. *Athlete's Edge: Faster, Quicker, Stronger with Vitamin D.* No city/state: Here and Now Books, 2011.

Carlson, Laurie Winn. *The Sunlight Solution: Why More Sun Exposure and Vitamin D are Essential to Your Health.* Amherst, NY: Prometheus, 2009.

Congressional Hearing, 93rd Congress, 1st Session, October 29-31, 1973: "Vitamin, Mineral, and Diet Supplements." Washington, D.C.: U.S. Government Printing Office, 1974.

Daniel, Esther Peterson, and Hazel Edith Munsell. *Vitamin Content of Foods.* Washington, D.C.: U.S. Government Printing Office, 1937.

Dowd, James E., and Diane Stafford. *The Vitamin D Cure.* Nashville, TN: Trade Paper Press, 2012.

Feldman, David (ed.). *Vitamin D: Volume 2: Health, Disease and Therapeutics.* London, UK: Academic Press, 2018.

Feltman, John (ed.). *Prevention's Food and Nutrition: The Most Complete Book Ever Written on Using Food and Vitamins to Fell Healthy and Cure Disease.* Emmaus, PA: Rodale Press,1993.

Giustina, A., and J. P. Bilezikian (eds.). *Vitamin D in Clinical Medicine.* London, UK: Karger, 2018.

God-Given Remedies for Everyday Ailments: 1,001 Amazing Secrets for Seniors That Prevent and Reverse Disease—Naturally. Peachtree City, GA: FC&A Medical Publishing, 2017.

Goldberg, Jane, with Jay Gutierrez. *The Hormesis Effect: The Miraculous Healing Power of Radioactive Stones.* Springhill, TN: Sea Raven Press, 2014.

Gombart, Adrian F. (ed.). *Vitamin D: Oxidative Stress, Immunity, and Aging.* Boca Raton, FL: CRC Press, 2013.

Guinness, Alma E. (ed.). *Great Health Hints and Handy Tips: More Than 4,000 Ideas to Help You Look and Feel Your Best.* Pleasantville, NY: Reader's Digest, 1994.

Hausman, Patricia, and Judith Benn Hurley. *The Healing Foods: The Ultimate Authority on the Curative Power of Nutrition.* Emmaus, PA: Rodale Press,1989.

Henriques, Tiago. *How Not To Die With True High-Dose Vitamin D Therapy: Coimbra's Protocol and the Secrets of Safe High-Dose Vitamin D3 and Vitamin K2 Supplementation.* Sao Paolo, Brazil: self-published, 2018.

Hessler, Margaret Constance. *Experiments Upon the Quantitative Differentiation of Vitamins A and D.* New York: Columbia University, 1926.

Holick, Michael F. *The Vitamin D Solution: A 3-Step Strategy to Cure Our Most Common Health Problems.* New York: Plume, 2011.

Hyde, P. J. *Sunlight, Vitamin D, and Prostate Cancer Risk: With References to Breast Cancer and Colon Cancer.* Bloomington, IN: Xlibris Corporation, 2004.

Kaplan, Gary, and Donna Beech. *Total Recovery: Solving the Mystery of Chronic Pain and Depression.* New York: Rodale, 2014.

Kennedy Jr., Robert F. *A Letter to Liberals: Censorship and COVID: An Attack on Science and American Ideals.* New York: Skyhorse Publishing, 2022.

——. *The Wuhan Cover-Up: And the Terrifying Bioweapons Arms Race.* New York: Skyhorse Publishing, 2023.

——. *Vax-Unvax: Let the Science Speak.* New York: Skyhorse Publishing, 2023.

Khalsa, Soram. *The Vitamin D Revolution: How the Power of This Amazing Vitamin Can Change Your Life.* Carlsbad, CA: Hay House, 2009.

Law, Jacky. *Big Pharma: Exposing the Global Healthcare Agenda.* New York: Carroll and Graf, 2006.

Litwack, Gerald (ed.). *Vitamin D Hormone.* London, UK: Academic Press, 2016.

Manning, John Ruel, E. M. Nelson, and Chester D. Tolle. *Vitamin D in Menhaden Fish Oils.* Washington, D.C.: U.S. Government Printing Office, 1931.

Mercola, Joseph. *Dark Deception: Discover the Truth About the Benefits of Sunlight Exposure.* Nashville, TN: Thomas Nelson, 2008.

——. *The Truth About COVID-19: Exposing The Great Reset, Lockdowns, Vaccine Passports, and the New Normal.* White River Junction, VT: Chelsea Green Publishing, 2021.

Mish, Frederick (ed.). *Webster's Ninth New Collegiate Dictionary.* 1828. Springfield, MA: Merriam-Webster, 1984 ed.

Murray, Frank. *Sunshine and Vitamin D: A Comprehensive Guide to the Benefits of the "Sunshine Vitamin."* Laguna Beach, CA: Basic Health Publications, 2008.

Norman, A. W., K. Schaefer, H. G. Grigoleit, and D. V. Herrath (eds.). *Vitamin D: Molecular, Cellular and Clinical Endocrinology.* Berlin, Germany: Walter de Gruyter, 1988.

Paul, Rand. *Deception: The Great Covid Cover-Up.* Washington, D.C.: Regnery Publishing, 2023.

Pludowski, Pawel, William B. Grant, Jerzy Konstantynowicz, and Michael F. Holick (eds.). *Classic and Pleiotropic Actions of Vitamin D.* Lausanne, Switzerland: Frontiers Media, 2007-2019.

Posner, Gerald. *Pharma: Greed, Lies, and the Poisoning of America.* New York: Simon and Schuster, 2021.

Proceedings of the Third Race Betterment Conference, January 2-6, 1928, pp. 609-639. Battle Creek, MI: The Race Betterment Foundation, 1928.

Ramavat, Sudha, and L. G. Ramavat. *Insight to Vitamin D: Miraculous Gift of Sun to All Beings.* New Delhi, India: Blue Rose One, 2023.

Recommended Dietary Allowances. Washington, D.C.: National Research Council, U.S. Food and Nutrition Board, 1941.

Reichrath, Jörg (ed.). *Sunlight, Vitamin D and Skin Cancer.* Cham, Switzerland: Springer, 2008-2020.

Ryan, Susan Rex. *Defend Your Life: Vitamin D3, a Safe, Easy, and Inexpensive Approach to Improving Quality of Life.* No city/state: Smilin Sue Publishing, 2013.

Schelle, Harald. *Vitamin D3 High Dosage: The Alternative to the Previous Therapy of Glaucoma.* Berlin, Germany: Epubli, 2018.

Seabrook, Lochlainn. *Victorian Hernia Cures: Nonsurgical Self-Treatment of Inguinal Hernia.* Springhill, TN: Sea Raven Press, 2022.

Somerville, Judson. *Optimal Dose: Restore Your Health With the Power of Vitamin D3.* Laredo, TX: Big Bend Press, 2018.

Stiebeling, Hazel Katherine. *Studies of the Relation of Vitamin D to the Deposition of Calcium in the Bones of Experimental Animals With Special Reference to the Quantitative Determination of Vitamin D.* New York: self-published, 1928.

Stolzt, Veronica D. (ed.). *Vitamin D: New Research.* New York: Nova Science, 2006.

"Symposium on Cod Liver Oil Presented." *The Pharmaceutical Era,* Vol. 60, May 30, 1925, pp. 675-677.

Your Body Can Heal Itself: Over 87 Foods Everyone Should Eat. Peachtree City, GA: FC&A Medical Publishing, 2008.

Vitamin, Mineral, and Diet Supplements. Washington, D.C.: U.S. Government Printing Office, 1973.

Watson, Ronald Ross (ed.). *Handbook of Vitamin D in Human Health: Prevention, Treatment and Toxicity.* Wageningen, Netherlands: Wageningen Academic Publishers, 2013.

Weiss, Suzanne E. (ed.) *Foods That Harm, Foods That Heal: An A-Z Guide to Safe and Healthy Eating.* Pleasantville, NY: Reader's Digest, 1997.

Zaidi, Sarfraz. *The Essential Role of Vitamin D: All You Need to Know About Vitamin D.* Troutdale, OR: self-published, 2024.

Zmijewski, Michal (ed.). *Vitamin D and Human Health.* Basel, Switzerland: MDPI, 2019.

INDEX

INCLUDES TOPICS, PEOPLE, KEYWORDS, KEY PHRASES, & SPELLING VARIATIONS
(Note: Some page numbers direct to endnotes on those particular pages rather than the pages themselves.)

animal products, 20, 22
animals, 41, 153
animals, and vitamin D, 41
ankles, clicking, popping, or cracking, 48
ankles, easily sprained, 48
ankylosing spondylitis, 48
Annunzio, Frank, 87
anorexia nervosa, 48
Antarctica, 175
anti-toxin mineral, 20, 33
antibodies, 55
antimicrobial, 21
antioxidant-rich foods, 77
antiphospholipid syndrome, 48
antisocial personality disorder, 48
antiviral, 21
anti-inflammatory, 21
anxiety, 48, 49, 56, 62, 63, 65, 70
aortic aneurysm, 47, 48
APD, 48
aphthous stomatitis, 48, 66
apoptosis, 21
Appalachia, 175
appendicitis, 48
appetite, reduced or loss of, 48
APS, 48
arbitrary limits, set by FDA, 84
ARDS, 47, 48
arms, 34, 36, 73, 153
arrhythmogenic right ventricular dysplasia, 48
arterial disease, 48, 65
arterial thrombosis, 48
arthritic pain, 77
arthritis, 21, 41, 48, 67, 68, 77
ascorbic acid, 18, 19
ASD, 48, 49
Asperger's syndrome, 48
aspergillosis, 48
asthma, 48
astronomy, 175
asymptomatic, 45
ataxia, 48
atherosclerosis, 48, 57
athletes' foot, 48
athletic performance, 48
Atkins, Chet, 175
ATL, 47
atopic dermatitis, 49
atopic eczema, 49
atrial fibrillation, 48, 49
atrial heart septal defect, 49
attack, 57, 71, 153
attention-deficit disorder, 49
attention-deficit/hyperactivity disorder, 47, 49
autism, 49
autistic spectrum disorder, 48, 49

auto brewery syndrome, 49
autoimmune diseases, 28
autoimmune health, 21
autoimmune thyroiditis, 49
autoimmune-inflammatory diseases, 49, 61, 69, 70
avocado oil, 77
avocados, 18, 36
babesiosis, 49
back, 6, 15, 36, 45, 46, 49, 61
back pain (lower), 49
bacterial infections, 49
bacterial origin, 18
bacterial vaginosis, 49
Barakat syndrome, 49, 57
basal cell nevus syndrome, 49
battle, 153
Bazex-Dupré-Christol syndrome, 49
BCNS, 49
BDD, 49
beach, 153
Becker, Karen, 41
beef liver, 32
behavior, 48, 49, 52, 68, 69
Behcet's disease, 49
benign mesothelioma, 49
benign paroxysmal positional vertigo, 49, 50
benign prostate enlargement, 49
benign tumor, 66
bent bones, 49
Berardinelli-Seip congenital lipodystrophy, 49
Berg, Eric, 22, 23, 27, 37
Bible, 78, 175, 177
BID, 50
Big Pharma, 31
bile duct cancer, 49, 51
binge eating, 49
bioassays, 174
bioavailability, 37
bioavailability, of vitamin D, 37
biochemistry, 40
biography, 2, 175
biological health, 21
biomedical research, 33
bipolar disorder, 49
birds, 41
birds, and vitamin D, 41
birth, 33
bladder cancer, 49, 72
bladder infections, 49
bleached foods, 33
blindness, 49
blocked arteries, 49
blood, 11, 22, 29, 35, 36, 39, 40, 44, 49, 57-59, 63, 80, 173
blood cancers, 49
blood clotting, 49

sea, 5, 6, 77, 152, 153, 179, 181
Sea Raven Press, 5, 6, 152, 153, 179, 181
sea salt, 77
Seabrook, Lochlainn, 2, 3, 16, 153, 175, 181
season, 30, 33, 73
seasonal affective disorder, 68, 69
seasonal allergic conjunctivitis, 69
seborrhoeic keratosis, 69
secosteroid hormone, 23
secosterols, 174
seed, 77
seed oils, 77
seeds, 18, 76
seizures, 40, 55, 67
selective mutism, 69
self-diagnostic experiments, 16
self-harm, 69
self-help, 2
seniors, 33, 34, 152
sensitivity to pain, increased, 69
sensorineural deafness, 49, 57, 69
sepsis, 69
septic shock, 69
services, 13, 14, 65, 174
severe acute respiratory syndrome, 68, 69
sex addiction, 52, 69
shared delusional disorder, 69
shiitake mushrooms, 32
shingles, 58, 69
short bowel syndrome, 69
short QT syndrome, 69
shortness of breath, 69
SIADH, 69, 70
sick sinus syndrome, 69
sickle cell anemia, 69
sickle cell disease, 69
sideroblastic anemia, 69
SIDS, 69, 70
silent killer, vitamin D deficiency as a, 44
sinusitis, 69
sisters, 175
sitocalciferol, 20
Sjögren syndrome, 69
Skaggs, Ricky, 175
skin, 16, 21, 22, 30, 33-36, 40, 55, 62, 64-66, 69, 73, 153
skin cancer, 34, 35, 62, 64, 69, 153
skin cancer (melanoma), 69
skin cancer (non-melanoma), 69
skin cancer, fear of, 34
skin color, 16, 30, 40
skin conditions, 69
skin damage, and tanning beds, 36
skin infections, 69
skin light sensitivity, 66, 69

skin melanin content, 33
skin tags, 69
slapped cheek syndrome, 55, 69
SLE, 61, 69, 70
sleep, 29, 47, 52, 53, 60, 64, 68, 69
sleep apnea, 64, 69
sleep issues, 69
sleep terrors, 64, 69
sleep, poor quality, 69
sleepwalking, 69
smallpox, 69
smell impairment, 70
Smith-Lemli-Opitz-syndrome, 68, 70
smog, 33
smoking, 64, 70, 76
snacking, 77
snakes, 41
snakes, and vitamin D, 41
social anxiety disorder, 70
soft drinks, 76
soft tissue, 40, 70
soft tissue sarcomas, 70
solanine, 77
soldiers, 175
somatization disorder, 70
Sons of Confederate Veterans, 175
sore throat, 70
sound waves, 57
South, 2, 93, 175, 177
South Dakota, 93
spasmodic dysphonia, 61, 70
spasms, 70
spices, 76, 77
spicy foods, 78
spinach, 76
spinal cord disease, 70
spinal cord injury, 70
spiritual guidance, 78
spiritual healers, 78
spiritual leaders, 78
spleen issues, 70
stainless steel cookware, 76
staphylococcus aureus, 70
starchy vegetables, 18
Steck Report, 28
Stephens, Alexander H., 175
sternum, pain on touching, 70
steroids, 19, 62
sterols, 19
stillbirth, 70
Still's syndrome (or disease), 70
stomach, 37, 70
stomach ache, 70
stomach cancer, 70
stomach ulcer, 70
storage, 57, 89, 96
strange disorders, 16
streptococcus pyogenes, 70
stress, 27, 37, 52, 53, 67, 74, 78, 152

KEYS & METRIC MEASURE CONVERSION TABLES RELATED SPECIFICALLY TO VITAMIN D

BLOOD LEVEL OF 25 (OH) VITAMIN D CONVERSION TABLE

➡ ng: nanogram
➡ ml: milliliter
➡ nmol: nanomole
➡ L: liter

1 ng/ml = 2.5 nmol/L
30 ng/ml = 75 nmol/L
100 ng/ml = 250 nmol/L
(Source: Zaidi, p. 244)

VITAMIN D DOSAGE CONVERSION TABLE

➡ IU: International Unit is a measure of biological activity and is
   different for each substance.
➡ mcg (also written μg): microgram, is one millionth of one
   gram. [As of 2016 this is the new measurement for vitamin D.]
➡ mg: milligram, is one thousandth of one gram.

To convert one IU of vitamin D to mcg, multiply the IU by 0.025.
This formula gives the following measurements:

1 IU = 0.025 mcg (or 0.00003 mg)
40 IU = 1 mcg (or 0.001 mg)
100 IU = 2.5 mcg (or 0.003 mg)
200 IU = 5 mcg (or 0.005 mg)
400 IU = 10 mcg (or 0.010 mg)
500 IU = 12.5 mcg (or 0.01 mg)
800 IU = 20 mcg (or 0.02 mg)
1000 IU = 25 mcg (or 0.03 mg)
2000 IU = 50 mcg (or 0.05 mg)
5000 IU = 125 mcg (or 0.13 mg)
10,000 IU = 250 mcg (or 0.25 mg)
50,000 IU = 1,250 mcg (or 1.25 mg)
100,000 IU = 2,500 mcg (or 2.5 mg)
200,000 IU = 5,000 mcg (or 5 mg)
300,000 IU = 7,500 mcg (or 7.5 mg)
500,000 IU = 12,500 mcg (or 12.5 mg)
(Source: U.S. government, FDA)

NEW 2016 FDA LABELING REGULATIONS
FOR MANUFACTURERS OF RETAIL FOOD PRODUCTS

"In 2016, the FDA amended the regulations for the nutrition labeling of conventional foods and dietary supplements to include updated Daily Values (DV), as Reference Daily Intakes (RDIs), for folate, niacin, vitamin A, vitamin D, and vitamin E. These RDIs are based on the Dietary Reference Intakes (DRIs), specifically Recommended Dietary Allowances (RDAs) published by the National Academy of Medicine (NAM, formerly known as the Institute of Medicine (IOM)). Except for niacin, which had its unit of measure established in the 1989 RDA as "Niacin Equivalent," the other four nutrients have new units of measure associated with the updated RDAs established by the NAM.

"Vitamin D, also known as calciferol, comprises a group of fat-soluble secosterols where the two major forms are vitamin D2 (ergocalciferol) and vitamin D3 (cholecalciferol). One IU of vitamin D has been previously defined as the activity of 0.025 mcg of cholecalciferol (Vitamin D3) in bioassays with rats and chicks:

$$1 \text{ mcg cholecalciferol} = 40 \text{ IU vitamin D}$$

"Vitamin D is considered a nutrient of public health significance, and so mandatory declaration of vitamin D is necessary to assist consumers in maintaining healthy dietary practices (81 FR 33742 at 33891). The [new] required unit of measure for vitamin D is "mcg" for both conventional foods and dietary supplements. It is also permissible to include the voluntary labeling of vitamin D in IU, in parentheses, next to the mandatory declaration in mcg units (81 FR 33742 at 33912-33913)."

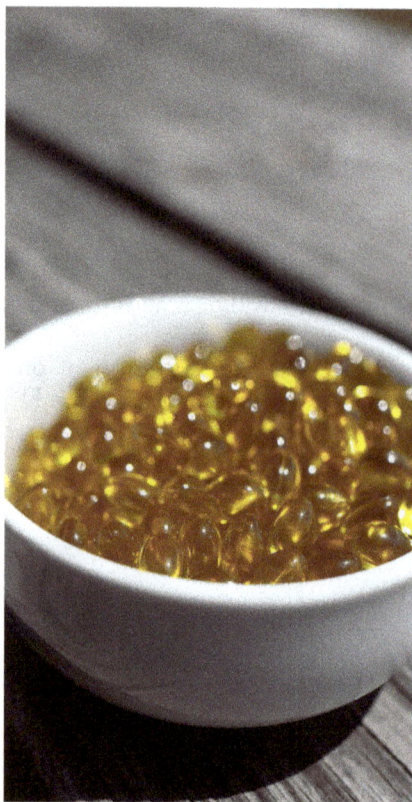

Photograph by Lochlainn Seabrook. Copyright © Lochlainn Seabrook.

(Source: "Guidance for Industry: Converting Units of Measure for Folate, Niacin, and Vitamins A, D, and E on the Nutrition and Supplement Facts Labels," U.S. Department of Health and Human Services, Food and Drug Administration, Center for Food Safety and Applied Nutrition, August 2019.)

MEET THE AUTHOR

NEO-VICTORIAN SCHOLAR LOCHLAINN SEABROOK, a descendant of the families of Alexander Hamilton Stephens, John Singleton Mosby, Edmund Winchester Rucker, and William Giles Harding, is a 7th generation Kentuckian and one of the most prolific and widely read writers in the world today. Known by literary critics as the "new Shelby Foote," the "American Robert Graves," and the "Southern Joseph Campbell," and by his fans as the "Voice of the Traditional South," he is a recipient of the United Daughters of the Confederacy's prestigious Jefferson Davis Historical Gold Medal, and is considered the foremost Southern interpreter of American Civil War history—or what he refers to as the War for the Constitution (1861-1865). A lifelong nonfiction writer, the Sons of Confederate Veterans member has authored and edited books ranging in topics from history, politics, science, comparative religion, spirituality, astronomy, entertainment, military, biography, mysticism, photography, and Bible studies, to nature, technology, music, humor, gastronomy, etymology, onomastics, mysteries, alternative health, comparative mythology, genealogy, Christian history, diet and nutrition, and the paranormal; books that his readers describe as "game changers," "transformative," and "life altering."

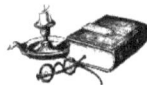

One of the world's most popular living historians, he is a 17th generation Southerner of Appalachian heritage who descends from dozens of patriotic Revolutionary War soldiers and Confederate soldiers from Kentucky, Tennessee, North Carolina, and Virginia. Also a history, wildlife, and nature preservationist, the well-respected polymath began life as a child prodigy, later maturing into an archetypal Renaissance Man. Besides being an accomplished and esteemed author, historian, biographer, creative, and Bible authority, the influential litterateur is also a Kentucky Colonel, eagle scout, entrepreneur, screenwriter, nature, wildlife, and landscape photographer and videographer, artist, graphic designer, content creator, genealogist, inventor, former history museum docent, and a former ranch hand, zookeeper, and wrangler. A songwriter (of some 3,000 songs in a dozen genres), he is also a film composer, multi-instrument musician, vocalist, session player, and music producer who has worked and performed with some of Nashville's top musicians and singers.

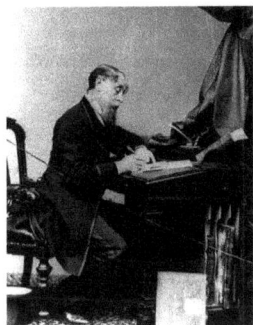

Currently Seabrook is the multi-genre author and editor of 100 adult and children's books (totaling some 30,000 pages and 15,000,000 words) that have earned him accolades from around the globe. His works, which have sold on every continent except Antarctica, have introduced hundreds of thousands to vital facts that have been left out of our mainstream books. He has been endorsed internationally by leading experts, museum curators, award-winning historians, bestselling authors, celebrities, filmmakers, noted scientists, well regarded educators, TV show hosts and producers, renowned military artists, venerable heritage organizations, and distinguished academicians of all races, creeds, and colors.

Of northern, western, and central European ancestry, he is the 6th great-grandson of the Earl of Oxford and a descendant of European royalty through his Kentucky father and West Virginia mother. His modern day cousins include: Johnny Cash, Elvis Presley, Lisa Marie Presley, Billy Ray and Miley Cyrus, Patty Loveless, Tim McGraw, Lee Ann Womack, Dolly Parton, Pat Boone, Naomi, Wynonna, and Ashley Judd, Ricky Skaggs, the Sunshine Sisters, Martha Carson, Chet Atkins, Patrick J. Buchanan, Cindy Crawford, Bertram Thomas Combs (Kentucky's 50th governor), Edith Bolling (second wife of President Woodrow Wilson), Andy Griffith, Riley Keough, George C. Scott, Robert Duvall, Reese Witherspoon, Lee Marvin, Rebecca Gayheart, and Tom Cruise.

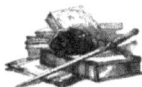

A constitutionalist, avid outdoorsman, and gun rights advocate, Seabrook is the author of the international blockbuster, *Everything You Were Taught About the Civil War is Wrong, Ask a Southerner!* He lives with his wife and family in the magnificent Rocky Mountains, heart of the American West, where you will find him hiking, filming, and writing.

For more information on author Mr. Seabrook visit

LOCHLAINNSEABROOK.COM

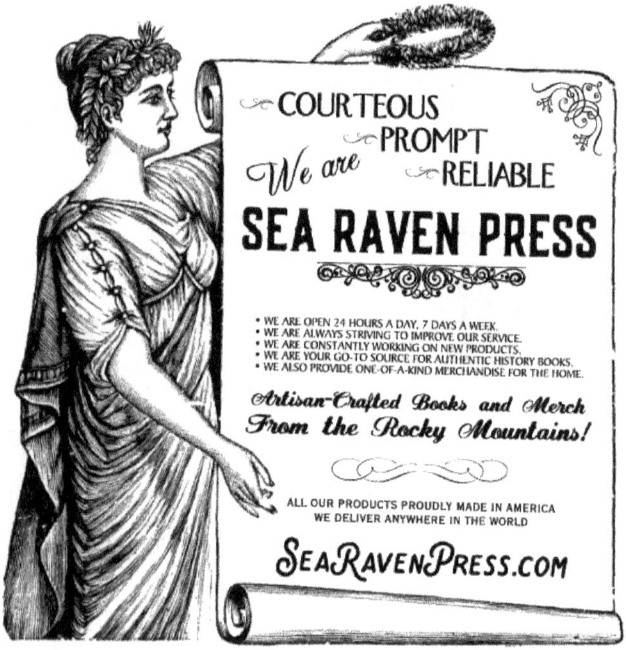
COURTEOUS
PROMPT
We are
RELIABLE
SEA RAVEN PRESS
• WE ARE OPEN 24 HOURS A DAY, 7 DAYS A WEEK.
• WE ARE ALWAYS STRIVING TO IMPROVE OUR SERVICE.
• WE ARE CONSTANTLY WORKING ON NEW PRODUCTS.
• WE ARE YOUR GO-TO SOURCE FOR AUTHENTIC HISTORY BOOKS.
• WE ALSO PROVIDE ONE-OF-A-KIND MERCHANDISE FOR THE HOME.
Artisan-Crafted Books and Merch
From the Rocky Mountains!
ALL OUR PRODUCTS PROUDLY MADE IN AMERICA
WE DELIVER ANYWHERE IN THE WORLD
SEARAVENPRESS.COM

★ "I love Lochlainn Seabrook's style and approach. It's not the 'norm.' What a miracle his books are. . . . He is a literal life changing author! Amazing books!" — KEITH PARISH

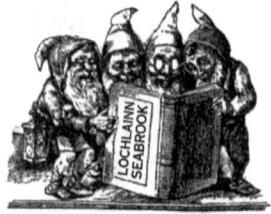

★ "I adore Mr. Seabrook's style and I love his books. I love an author that does proper research, and still finds a way to engage the reader. Mr. Seabrook does an admirable job of both." — DONALD CAUL

★ "Lochlainn Seabrook's books are much more well researched and authoritative than those eminently celebrated as being the authorities on the subjects he writes on. You can always trust to find the truth in his writings. . . . He does not rewrite history, but instead shows it as it is." — GARY STIER

★ "I love all of Colonel Seabrook's books. They are informative and enlightening, and his warm Southern hospitality writing style makes you feel right at home." — KEITH CRAVEN

★ "Lochlainn Seabrook's work is an absolute treasure of scholarship and historic scope." — MARK WAYNE CUNNINGHAM

★ "Mr. Seabrook's command of . . . history is breathtaking. . . . He deserves great renown—check out his books!" — MARGARET SIMMONS

★ "I love Seabrook's writings. LOVE!!! . . . So grateful to know the truth! Keep writing Lochlainn!!!" — REBECCA DALRYMPLE

★ "Lochlainn Seabrook . . . [has] probably [written] the best book on mental science in existence by a living author. Along with Thomas Troward, Emmet Fox, and Jack Addington, Mr. Seabrook is one of the top four mental science authors of all time, since biblical times." - IAN BARTON STEWART

★ "Glad I discovered Mr. Seabrook! . . . He writes eye opening books! Unbelievable the facts he unearths - and he backs it all up with truth, notes, footnotes, and bibliography! . . . He always amazes me! His books always see the whole picture. His timelines and bibliographies are incredible. He always provides carefully reasoned arguments! He's the best. To me I think he's better than the late great Shelby Foote! America needs more like Lochlainn Seabrook. I can't wait to own all of his books on the war someday. Everyone who wants the Truth, who seeks the Truth and wants the full story, should read his books." — JOHN BULL BADER

★ "I love all of Colonel Seabrook's books!" — DEBBIE SIDLE

★ "Lochlainn Seabrook is well educated and versed in what he writes and I'm impressed with the delivery." — THOMAS L. WHITE

★ "Thank you Lochlainn Seabrook for your wonderful books! You are the real deal! You are an amazing author and I love your books!!" — SOPHIA MEOW CELLIST

★ "I really enjoy Mr. Seabrook's books! His knowledge is beyond belief!" — SANDRA FISH

★ "Love Lochlainn Seabrook. Awesome!!" — ROBIN HENDERSON ARISTIDES

★ "Kudos to Lochlainn Seabrook who is a very good and informative professional truthful historian. We need more like him!" — AMY VACHON

Nurture Your Mind, Body, and Spirit!
READ THE BOOKS OF

SEA RAVEN PRESS

Visit our Webstore for a wide selection of wholesome, family-friendly, evidence-based, educational books for all ages. You'll be glad you did!

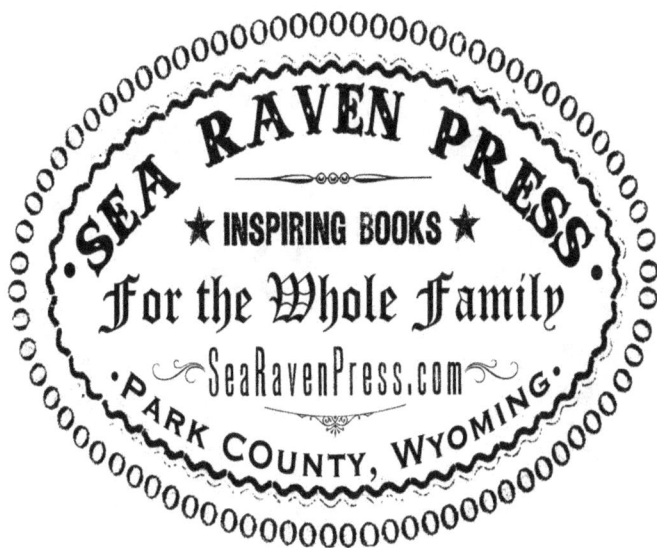

ARTISAN-CRAFTED BOOKS, MERCH, AND GIFTS FROM THE ROCKY MOUNTAINS!

SeaRavenPress.com
LochlainnSeabrook.com
TheBestCivilWarBookEver.com
AmbianceGoneWild.com
Pond5.com/artist/LochlainnSeabrook

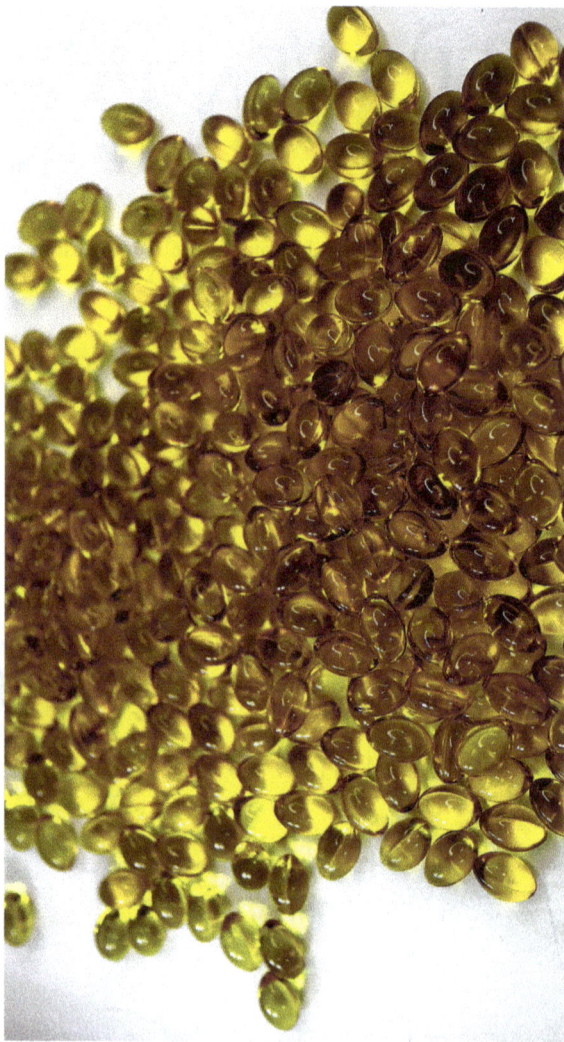

Photograph by Lochlainn Seabrook. Copyright © Lochlainn Seabrook.

If you enjoyed this book you will be interested in Colonel Seabrook's popular related title:

☛ VICTORIAN HERNIA CURES: NONSURGICAL SELF-TREATMENT OF INGUINAL HERNIA

Available from Sea Raven Press and wherever fine books are sold

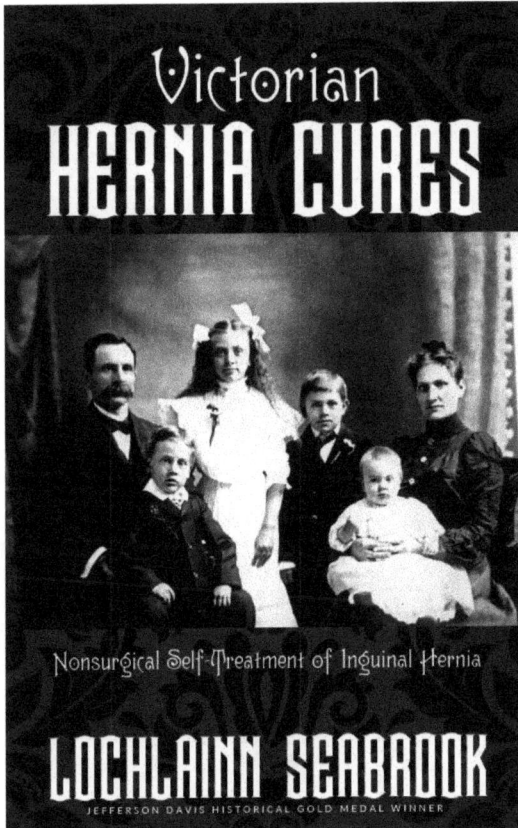

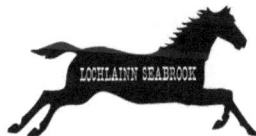

SeaRavenPress.com

www.ingramcontent.com/pod-product-compliance
Lightning Source LLC
Chambersburg PA
CBHW071126280326
41935CB00010B/1132